Decision modelling for health economic evaluation

D1202584

Handbooks in Health Economic Evaluation Series

Series Editors: Alastair Gray and Andrew Briggs

Forthcoming volumes in the series:

Economic evaluation in clinical trials
Henry A Glick, Jalpa A Doshi, Seema S Sonnad and Daniel Polsky

Decision modelling for health economic evaluation

Andrew Briggs
Lindsay Chair in Health Policy & Economic Evaluation,
Section of Public Health & Health Policy,
University of Glasgow, UK

Karl Claxton
Professor of Economics, Department of Economics
and Related Studies and Centre for Health Economics,
University of York, UK

Mark Sculpher
Professor of Health Economics, Centre for Health
Economics, University of York, UK

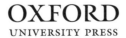
OXFORD
UNIVERSITY PRESS

OXFORD
UNIVERSITY PRESS

Great Clarendon Street, Oxford OX2 6DP

Oxford University Press is a department of the University of Oxford.
It furthers the University's objective of excellence in research, scholarship,
and education by publishing worldwide in

Oxford New York

Auckland Cape Town Dar es Salaam Hong Kong Karachi
Kuala Lumpur Madrid Melbourne Mexico City Nairobi
New Delhi Shanghai Taipei Toronto

With offices in

Argentina Austria Brazil Chile Czech Republic France Greece
Guatemala Hungary Italy Japan Poland Portugal Singapore
South Korea Switzerland Thailand Turkey Ukraine Vietnam

Oxford is a registered trade mark of Oxford University Press
in the UK and in certain other countries

Published in the United States
by Oxford University Press Inc., New York

British Library Cataloguing in Publication Data

Data available

Library of Congress Cataloging in Publication Data

Data available

Typeset in Minion
Printed in Great Britain
on acid-free paper by
Ashford colour press Ltd., Gosport, Hampshire

ISBN 978–0–19–852662–9 (Pbk.)

10 9 8 7 6 5

For Eleanor, Zoe and Clare

Preface

Decision Modelling for Health Economic Evaluation

"All models are wrong ... some are useful"

George Box

This book reflects the increasing demand for technical details of the use of decision models for health economic evaluation. The material presented in this book has evolved from a number of sources, but the style of presentation owes much to the three-day residential course on "Advanced Modelling Methods for Health Economic Evaluation" that has been running since September 2003, and which offered us the opportunity to try out the material on willing participants from a range of professional backgrounds. The book, like the course, remains essentially practical, the aim has always been to provide a help to analysts, perhaps struggling with modelling methods for the first time, by demonstrating exactly how things might be done. For this reason, many of the teaching examples, spreadsheet templates and solutions are provided in the book and on the accompanying website. We are indebted to a long list of course alumni who have helpfully ironed out many of the typos, errors and gremlins that are an inevitable consequence of producing such material.

In addition to the participants of the course itself, a number of people have been instrumental in checking and commenting on previous drafts of material at various stages of its development. Particular thanks must go to Elisabeth Fenwick, who has been a constant presence from the inception of the very first course and has commented from the very first draft of the course materials right through to the final version of the book. We would also like to thank Pelham Barton, Jonathon Karnon, Karen Kuntz, and Gillian Sanders for comments on specific chapters; Gemma Dunn and Garry Barton for checking exercises and proofs as part of the final stages of development; and finally Alastair Gray for comments and guidance in his role as series editor. Of course, remaining errors are our own responsibility.

Finally, in seeing the final version of the manuscript published, we are acutely aware of the fast-moving nature of the field. The opening quote was made in the 1970s in relation to statistical modelling of data, but we believe it applies just as well to decision modelling. The methods that we present in this book are just one way of looking at the world, it is not necessarily the correct way and there may well be other equally valid approaches to handle some of the issues we present as part of this book. Nevertheless, while future research will undoubtedly offer improvements on the techniques we propose here, we hope that the drawing together of this material in this form, if not entirely correct, will at least prove useful.

AB, KC & MS
May 2006

Series Preface

Economic evaluation in health care is a thriving international activity that is increasingly used to allocate scarce health resources, and within which applied and methodological research, teaching, and publication are flourishing. Several widely respected texts are already well-established in the market, so what is the rationale for not just one more book, but for a series? We believe that the books in the series *Handbooks in Health Economic Evaluation* share a strong distinguishing feature, which is to cover as much as possible of this broad field with a much stronger practical flavour than existing texts, using plenty of illustrative material and worked examples. We hope that readers will use this series not only for authoritative views on the current practice of economic evaluation and likely future developments, but for practical and detailed guidance on how to undertake an analysis. The books in the series are textbooks, but first and foremost they are handbooks.

Our conviction that there is a place for the series has been nurtured by the continuing success of two short courses we helped develop – Advanced Methods of Cost-Effectiveness Analysis, and Advanced Modelling Methods for Economic Evaluation. Advanced Methods was developed in Oxford in 1999 and has run several times a year ever since, in Oxford, Canberra and Hong Kong. Advanced Modelling was developed in York and Oxford in 2002 and has also run several times a year ever since, in Oxford, York, Glasgow and Toronto. Both courses were explicitly designed to provide computer-based teaching that would take participants through the theory but also the methods and practical steps required to undertake a robust economic evaluation or construct a decision-analytic model to current standards. The proof-of-concept was the strong international demand for the courses - from academic researchers, government agencies and the pharmaceutical industry – and the very positive feedback on their practical orientation.

So the original concept of the Handbooks series, as well as many of the specific ideas and illustrative material, can be traced to these courses. The Advanced Modelling course is in the phenotype of the first book in the series, *Decision Modelling for Health Economic Evaluation*, which focuses on the role and methods of decision analysis in economic evaluation. The Advanced Methods course has been an equally important influence on *Applied Methods of Cost-Effectiveness*, the third book in the series which sets out the key elements of analysing costs and outcomes, calculating cost-effectiveness and reporting results. The concept was then extended to cover several other important topic areas. First, the design, conduct and analysis of economic evaluations alongside clinical trials has become a specialised area of activity with distinctive methodological and practical issues, and its own debates and controversies. It seemed worthy of a dedicated volume, hence the second book in the series, *Economic Evaluation in Clinical Trials*. Next, while the use of cost-benefit analysis in health care has spawned a substantial literature, this is mostly theoretical, polemical, or focused on specific issues such as willingness to pay. We believe the fourth book in the series, *Applied Methods of Cost-Benefit Analysis in Health Care*, fills an important gap in the literature by providing a comprehensive guide to the theory but also the practical conduct of cost-benefit analysis, again with copious illustrative material and worked examples.

Each book in the series is an integrated text prepared by several contributing authors, widely drawn from academic centres in the UK, the United States, Australia and elsewhere. Part of our role as editors has been to foster a consistent style, but not to try to impose any particular line: that would have been unwelcome and also unwise amidst the diversity of an evolving field. News and information about the series, as well as supplementary material for each book, can be found at the series website: http://www.herc.ox.ac.uk/books

Alastair Gray   Andrew Briggs
Oxford   Glasgow
July 2006

Contents

Chapter 1

Introduction

Economic evaluation is increasingly used to inform the decisions of various health care systems about which health care interventions to fund from available resources. This is particularly true of decisions about the coverage or reimbursement of new pharmaceuticals. The first jurisdictions to use economic evaluation in this way were the public health systems in Australia and Ontario, Canada (Commonwealth Department of Health 1992; Ministry of Health 1994); since then many others have developed similar arrangements (Hjelmgren *et al.* 2001). In the UK, the National Institute for Health and Clinical Excellence (NICE) has a wider purview in terms of health technologies, and uses economic evaluation to inform decisions about medical devices, diagnostic technologies and surgical procedures, as well as pharmaceuticals (NICE 2004*a*). The ever-present need to allocate finite resources between numerous competing interventions and programmes means that economic evaluation methods are also used, to a greater or lesser degree, at 'lower levels' within many health care systems (Hoffmann *et al.* 2000).

The increasing use of economic evaluation for decision making has placed some very clear requirements on researchers in terms of analytic methods (Sculpher *et al.* 2005). These include the need to incorporate all appropriate evidence into the analysis, to compare new technologies with the full range of relevant alternative options and to reflect uncertainty in evidence in the conclusions of the analysis. The need to satisfy these requirements provides a strong rationale for decision analytic modelling as a framework for economic evaluation. This book focuses on the role and methods of decision analysis in economic evaluation. It moves beyond more introductory texts in terms of modelling methods (Drummond *et al.* 2005), but seeks to ground this exposition in the needs of decision making in collectively-funded health care systems. Through the use of a mixture of general principles, case studies and exercises, the book aims at providing a thorough understanding of the latest methods in this field, as well as insights into where these are likely to move over the next few years.

In this introductory chapter, we seek to provide a brief overview of the main tenets of economic evaluation in health care, the needs of decision making and the rationale for decision analytic modelling.

1.1. Defining economic evaluation

It is not the purpose of this book to provide a detailed introduction to economic evaluation in health care in general. Good introductory texts are available (Sloan 1995; Gold *et al.* 1996; Drummond *et al.* 2005), and we provide only an overview of the key aspects of these methods here.

Economic evaluation in health care can be defined as the comparison of alternative options in terms of their costs and consequences (Drummond *et al.* 2005). Alternative options refer to the range of ways in which health care resources can be used to increase population health; for example, pharmaceutical and surgical interventions, screening and health promotion programmes. In this book terms like 'options', 'technologies', 'programmes' and 'interventions' are used interchangeably. Health care costs refer to the value of tangible resources available to the health care system; for example, clinical and other staff, capital equipment and buildings, and consumables such as drugs. Non-health service resources are also used to produce health care, such as the time of patients and their families. Consequences represent all the effects of health care programmes other than those on resources. These generally focus on changes in individuals' health, which can be positive or negative, but can also include other effects that individuals may value, such as reassurance and information provision.

As is clear in the definition above, economic evaluation is strictly comparative. It is not possible to establish the economic value of one configuration of resources (e.g. the use of a particular medical intervention) unless its costs and consequences are compared with at least one alternative option.

1.2. Alternative paradigms for economic evaluation

It is possible to trace the disciplinary origins of economic evaluation back in several directions. One direction relates to welfare economic theory (Ng 1983) which implies that health care programmes should be judged in the same way as any other proposed change in resource allocation. That is, the only question is whether they represent a potential Pareto improvement in social welfare – could the gainers from a policy change compensate the losers and remain in a preferred position compared with before the change? In the context of resource allocation in health care, therefore, welfare theory does not have has an interest solely in whether policy changes improve health outcomes as measured, for example, on the basis of health-related quality of life (HRQL). There is also an implicit view that the current distribution of income is, if not optimal, then at least acceptable (Pauly 1995), and that the distributive impacts of health care programmes, and the failure actually to pay compensation, are negligible.

Cost-benefit analysis is the form of economic evaluation that springs from this theoretical paradigm, based on the concept of potential Pareto improvement (Sugden and Williams 1979). Cost-benefit analysis seeks to value the full range of health and other consequences of a policy change and compare this with resource costs as a form of compensation test. In health care, benefit valuation has usually been in the form of contingent valuation or willingness to pay methods (Johanesson 1995; Pauly 1995). This involves seeking individuals' valuation of the consequences of health care programmes in terms of hypothetical monetary payment to be paid to obtain a benefit or to avoid a disbenefit (Gafni 1991; Diener *et al.* 1998).

A second disciplinary origin for economic evaluation in health care is in operations research and management science. In general, this has taken the form of constrained maximization: the maximization of a given objective function subject to a set of constraints. However, it should be noted that this view of economic evaluation is also consistent with the concept of social decision making which has been described in the economics literature as an alternative to standard welfare theory (Sugden and Williams 1979). There has also been some development in economics of the concept of 'extra welfarism' as a normative framework for decision making (Culyer 1989). In essence, these non-welfarist perspectives take an exogenously defined societal objective and budget constraint for health care. Cost-effectiveness analysis (CEA) is the form of economic evaluation that has generally been used in health care to apply these principles of resource allocation. It is possible to justify CEA within a welfare theoretic framework (Garber and Phelps 1997; Meltzer 1997; Weinstein and Manning 1997), but generally it is the social decision making view that has implicitly or explicitly provided the methodological foundations of CEA in health.

1.3. **Cost-effectiveness analysis in health care**

There is debate about the appropriate normative theory for economic evaluation in health care. There can be little doubt, however, that some form of CEA predominates in terms of applied research in health (Pritchard 1998). In the context of health care, CEA would typically be characterized with a health-related objective function and constraints centred on a (narrow or broad) health care budget. There are many examples in the CEA literature which use measures of health specific to the disease or intervention under consideration. Examples of such measures are episode-free days (asthma) (Sculpher and Buxton 1993), true positive cases detected (breast cancer) (Bryan *et al.* 1995) and percentage reduction in blood cholesterol (coronary heart disease) (Schulman *et al.* 1990). However, given the need in most health care systems to make resource allocation decisions across a whole range of disease areas, CEA has increasingly been based on a single ('generic') measure of health. Although other measures have been suggested, the quality-adjusted life-year (QALY) is the most frequently used measure for this purpose.

The use of the QALY as the measure of effect in a CEA is often referred to as cost-utility analysis (Drummond *et al.* 2005). On the basis that health care programmes and interventions aim to impact on individuals' length of life and health-related quality of life, the QALY seeks to reflect these two aspects in a single measure. Various introductions to the QALY as used in CEA are available (Torrance and Feeny 1989; Drummond *et al.* 2005), as well as more detailed descriptions of the methods used to derive 'quality-weights' (often called values or utilities) (Torrance 1986; Patrick and Erickson 1993) and of the assumptions underlying QALYs (Pliskin *et al.* 1980; Loomes and McKenzie 1989). Despite its limitations, the QALY remains the only generic measure of health that has been used in a large range of clinical areas.

In some introductory texts on economic evaluation in health, and in a number of applied studies, cost-minimization analysis is described as a separate type of economic evaluation. This has been used under the assumption that effects (on health and other possible attributes) do not differ between the options under consideration. In such circumstances, the option with the lowest cost represents the greatest value for money. This is essentially a simplified CEA, but it has been criticized because, in many circumstances, the assumption of equal effects is based on an erroneous interpretation of a statistical hypothesis test and ignores the uncertainty which will invariably exist in the differential effects between options (Briggs and O'Brien 2001).

As mentioned earlier, the origin of CEA is generally seen to be in constrained optimization. In principle, the methods of identifying whether a particular technology is appropriate (i.e. cost-effective) would involve looking at each and every use of resources and selecting those which maximize the health-related objective function subject to the budget constraint (Stinnett and Paltiel 1996). The information needed to implement these methods in full, however, has so far made their practical use for decision making impossible. The result has been the use of simplified 'decision rules' for the identification of the most cost-effective option from among those being compared (Johannesson and Weinstein 1993). These are based on some simplifying assumptions, such as options generating constant returns to scale and being perfectly divisible (Birch and Gafni 1992).

Standard cost-effectiveness decision rules involve relating differences in costs between options under comparison to differences in benefits. In the case of an option being dominant (costing less and generating greater effects than all the alternatives with which it is being compared), it is unequivocally cost-effective. However, if an option generates additional benefits but at extra cost it can still be considered cost-effective. In such a situation, the option's incremental costs and effects are calculated and compared with those of other uses of health service resources. For example, if a new drug therapy for Alzheimer's disease is found to generate more QALYs than currently available treatment options, but also to add to costs, then a decision to fund the new therapy will involve opportunity costs falling on the health care system (i.e. the QALYs forgone from programmes or interventions which are removed or down-scaled to fund the new drug). The analytical question is whether the QALYs generated from the new Alzheimer's therapy are greater than the opportunity costs. Given limited information on the costs and effects associated with the full range of uses of health service resources, simplified decision rules have centred on the calculation of an incremental cost-effectiveness ratio (ICER); that is, the additional cost per extra unit of effect (e.g. QALY) from the more effective treatment. When the ICER is compared with those of other interventions, or with some notional threshold value which decision makers are (assumed to be) willing to pay for an additional unit of effect, the preferred option from those being evaluated can be established. A further concept in decision rules is 'extended dominance'. This can occur when three or more options are being compared and is present when an option has a higher ICER than a more effective comparator. This concept is described further in the next chapter.

1.4. The role of decision analysis in economic evaluation

Decision analysis represents a set of analytic tools that are quite distinct from cost-benefit analysis and CEA but can be seen as complementary to both. Decision analysis has been widely used in a range of disciplines including business analysis and engineering (Raiffa and Schlaifer 1959). In health care, it is an established framework to inform decision making under conditions of uncertainty (Weinstein and Fineberg 1980; Sox *et al.* 1988; Hunink *et al.* 2001). Decision analysis has been used more generally in health care evaluation than in economic evaluation, in terms of informing clinical decisions at population and individual levels (McNeil *et al.* 1976; Schoenbaum *et al.* 1976; Gottlieb and Pauker 1981).

Basic concepts in decision modelling for CEA have been covered elsewhere (Hunink *et al.* 2001; Drummond *et al.* 2005). Here we summarize some of the key concepts and principles in the area.

1.4.1. What is decision modelling?

Decision analysis has been defined as a systematic approach to decision making under uncertainty (Raiffa 1968). In the context of economic evaluation, a decision analytic model uses mathematical relationships to define a series of possible consequences that would flow from a set of alternative options being evaluated. Based on the inputs into the model, the likelihood of each consequence is expressed in terms of probabilities, and each consequence has a cost and an outcome. It is thus possible to calculate the expected cost and expected outcome of each option under evaluation. For a given option, the expected cost (outcome) is the sum of the costs (outcomes) of each consequence weighted by the probability of that consequence.

A key purpose of decision modelling is to allow for the variability and uncertainty associated with all decisions. The concepts of variability and uncertainty are developed later in the book (particularly in Chapter 4). The way a decision model is structured will reflect the fact that the consequences of options are variable. For example, apparently identical patients will respond differently to a given intervention. This might be characterized in terms, for example, of dichotomous events such as 'response' and 'no response' to treatment. The model will be structured to reflect the fact that, for an individual patient, whether or not they respond will be unknown in advance. The like-lihood of a response will be expressed as a probability, which is a parameter to the model. However, the estimation of this parameter is uncertain and this should also be allowed for in the model using sensitivity analysis.

As a vehicle for economic evaluation, the 'decision' relates to a range of resource allocation questions. Examples of these include: Should a collectively-funded health system fund a new drug for Alzheimer's disease? What is the most cost-effective diagnostic strategy for suspected urinary tract infection in children? Would it represent a good use of our limited resources to undertake additional research regarding one or more parameters in our decision model?

1.4.2. The role of decision modelling for economic evaluation

Decision analysis has had a controversial role in economic evaluation in health care (Sheldon 1996; Buxton *et al.* 1997). However, the growing use of economic evaluation to inform specific decision problems facing health care decision makers (Hjelmgren *et al.* 2001) has seen an increased prominence for decision modelling as a vehicle for evaluation. The strongest evidence for this is probably the 2004 methods guidelines from the National Institute for Clinical Excellence in the UK (NICE 2004b), but it is also apparent with other decision makers.

In part, the increasing use of modelling in this context can be explained by the required features of any economic evaluation seeking to inform decision making. The key requirements of such studies are considered below.

Synthesis

It is essential for economic evaluation studies to use all relevant evidence. In the context of parameters relating to the effectiveness of interventions, this is consistent with a central tenet of evidence-based medicine (Sackett *et al.* 1996). However, it should also apply to other parameters relevant to economic evaluation, such as resource use and quality-of-life weights (utilities). Rarely will all relevant evidence come from a single source and, typically, it will have to be drawn from a range of disparate sources. A framework is, therefore, needed within which to synthesize this range of evidence. This needs to provide a structure in which evidence can be brought to bear on the decision problem. Hence it should provide a means to characterize the natural history of a given condition, the impact of alternative interventions and the costs and health effects contingent on clinical events. This framework will also include the relationship between any intermediate clinical measure of effect and the ultimate measure of health gain required for CEA (Drummond *et al.* 2005).

Consideration of all relevant comparators

The cost-effectiveness of a given technology, programme or intervention can only be achieved in comparison with all alternative options that could feasibly be used in practice. These alternatives could relate to different sequences of treatments and/or stop-go decision rules on intervention. In most instances, a single study, such as a randomized trial, will not compare all alternatives relevant to the economic evaluation. There will, therefore, be a need to bring together data from several clinical studies using appropriate statistical synthesis methods (Sutton and Abrams 2001; Ades *et al.* 2006). Again, the decision model provides the framework to bring this synthesis to bear on the decision problem.

Appropriate time horizon

For decision making, economic evaluation requires that studies adopt a time horizon that is sufficiently long to reflect all the key differences between options in terms of costs and effects. For many interventions, this will effectively require a lifetime time horizon. This is particularly true of interventions with a potential mortality effect, where life expectancy calculations require full survival curves to be estimated. Economic evaluations based on a single source of patient-level data (e.g. a randomized trial or observational study) will rarely have follow-up which is sufficiently long to facilitate a lifetime time horizon. Again, the decision model becomes the framework within which to structure the extrapolation of costs and effects over time. There are two elements to this. The first relates to extending baseline costs and effects beyond the primary data source, where this may relate to natural history or one of the 'standard' therapies being evaluated (i.e. baseline effects). The second element concerns the continuation of the treatment effect; that is, the effectiveness of the interventions being evaluated relative to the baseline.

Uncertainty

A key requirement of economic evaluation for decision making is to indicate how uncertainty in the available evidence relating to a given policy problem translates into decision uncertainty; that is, the probability that a given decision is the correct one. A key objective of this book is to show how probabilistic decision models can fully account for this uncertainty, present this to decision makers and translate this into information about the value and optimal design of additional research.

1.4.3. Models versus trials

The importance of the randomized controlled trial in generating evidence for the evaluation of health care programmes and interventions has seen it develop a role as a vehicle for economic evaluation. That is, the trial provides the sole source of evidence on resource use and health effects that, together with external valuation data (in the form of unit costs and utilities), forms the basis of the estimate of cost-effectiveness. It has been well recognized that many trials exhibit weaknesses when used in this way, particularly 'regulatory trials' designed to support licensing applications for new pharmaceuticals (Drummond and Davies 1991). As noted previously, this includes the limited number of comparisons, short follow-up and a failure to collect all the evidence needed to address cost-effectiveness. As a result of these limitations, there has been extensive consideration of the appropriate design and analysis of trials for economic evaluation – these have variously been termed pragmatic or 'real world' studies (Freemantle and Drummond 1997; Coyle *et al.* 1998; Thompson and Barber 2000).

A large proportion of economic evaluation studies could be described as trial-based economic evaluations: since 1994, approximately 30 per cent of published economic evaluations on the NHS Economic Evaluation Database have been based on data from a single trial (www.york.ac.uk/inst/crd). Given the requirements of decision making described in the last section, however – in particular, the need to include all relevant evidence and compare all appropriate options – the appropriate role for an economic study based on a single trial, rather than a decision model, remains a source of debate.

1.5. **Summary and structure of the book**

This introductory chapter provides an overview of the key concepts behind economic evaluation of health care in general, and the role of decision analysis in this context. It has described the alternative theoretical origins lying behind economic evaluation – welfare economic theory and extra-welfarist approaches including social decision making. These alternative paradigms largely explain the existence of competing evaluation methods in economic evaluation – cost-benefit analysis and cost-effectiveness analysis – although the latter predominates in the applied literature. The role of decision analysis in economic evaluation can be seen as independent of either of these types of evaluation although it can complement both approaches. Within the social decision making paradigm, the requirements of decision making regarding resource allocation decisions emphasize the value of decision models. In particular, the need to synthesize all relevant evidence and to compare all options over an appropriate time horizon necessitates the need for a decision analytical framework.

In the remainder of this book, we develop further the methods of decision analysis for economic evaluation. Chapter 2 focuses on the cohort model and, in particular, the Markov model, a widely used form of decision model in CEA. Chapter 3 considers a range of possible extensions to the standard Markov model including reflecting time dependency and the use of patient-level simulations. Chapter 4 describes the methods for handling uncertainty in decision models, in particular, the use of probabilistic sensitivity analysis to reflect parameter uncertainty. Chapter 5 shows how decision uncertainty and heterogeneity in a model can be presented to decision makers using methods such as cost-effectiveness acceptability curves. Chapter 6 builds on the concepts in earlier chapters to show how probabilistic decision models can be used to quantify the cost of decision uncertainty and hence the value of additional information as a basis for research prioritization. Chapter 7 extends the value-of-information methods by looking at how probabilistic decision models can be used to identify the most efficient design of future research studies. Chapter 8 draws together the key conclusions from the preceding chapters.

1.6. **Exercises**

One of the features of this book is the emphasis on practical exercises that are designed to illustrate the application of many of the key issues covered in each chapter. These exercises are integrated into Chapters 2–6 and are based around the development of two example models, building in sophistication as the book progresses. The first example is a replication of a previously published model of combination therapy for HIV/AIDS (Chancellor *et al.* 1997), which, although somewhat out of date in terms of the treatment under evaluation, nevertheless represents a useful example that serves to illustrate a number of general modelling issues. The second example is a slightly simplified version of a model examining the cost-effectiveness of a new cemented hip prosthesis compared with the standard prosthesis that has been used in the NHS for many years (Briggs *et al.* 2004). The practical exercises are facilitated by a series of Microsoft Excel™ templates that set out the structure of the exercise and a set of solutions for each exercise. In most cases the templates in one chapter are based on the solution for the preceding chapter, such that the exercises build to a comprehensive evaluation of the decision problem.

It is worth being clear why we have chosen to use Excel as a platform for the exercises and recommend it more widely for undertaking cost-effectiveness modelling. Firstly, Excel is the most popular example of spreadsheet software (much of what we cover in the exercises is directly transferable to other spreadsheet packages). Although there are a number of good dedicated decision analysis packages available, in our experience none is capable of all the functions and presentation aspects of many full health economic models. Furthermore, where some functions are available (such as the ability to correlate parameters) the application can become something of a 'black box' – it is always worth knowing how to implement such methods from first principles. There are also a number of popular 'add-ins' for Excel, such as Crystal Ball and @Risk. These programs add to the functionality of Excel, particularly in relation to simulation methods. While these are much less of a black box, in that they can be employed to complement existing spreadsheet models, there is a problem in that models built with these add-ins can only be used by other people with the add-in software. This can severely limit the potential user base for a model. For these reasons we have chosen to demonstrate how the basic Excel package can be used for the complete modelling process. This has the advantage that the exercises are concerned with implementing the methods from first principles rather than coaching the reader in the use of software to implement the methods. That said, some basic familiarity with Excel operations is assumed.

A website for the book has been set up to give the reader access to the Excel templates that form the basis of the exercises. The web address is www.herc.ox.ac.uk/books/modelling.html and contains links to the exercise templates labelled by exercise number together with the solution files.

References

Ades, A. E., Sculpher, M. J., Sutton, A., Abrams, K., Cooper, N., Welton, N., *et al.* (2006) 'Bayesian methods for evidence synthesis in cost-effectiveness analysis', *PharmacoEconomics* 24: 1–19.

Birch, S. and Gafni, A. (1992) 'Cost effectiveness/utility analyses: do current decision rules lead us to where we want to be?', *Journal of Health Economics*, 11: 279–296.

Briggs, A. H. and O'Brien, B. J. (2001) 'The death of cost-minimisation analysis?', *Health Economics*, 10: 179–184.

Briggs, A., Sculpher, M., Dawson, J., Fitzpatrick, R., Murray, D. and Malchau, H. (2004) 'Are new cemented prostheses cost-effective? A comparison of the Spectron and the Charnley'. *Applied Health Economics & Health Policy*, 3(2): 78–89.

Bryan, S., Brown, J. and Warren, R. (1995) 'Mammography screening: an incremental cost-effectiveness analysis of two-view versus one-view procedures in London', *Journal of Epidemiology and Community Health*, 49: 70–78.

Buxton, M. J., Drummond, M. F., Van Hout, B. A., Prince, R. L., Sheldon, T. A., Szucs, T. and Vray, M. (1997) 'Modelling in economic evaluation: an unavoidable fact of life', *Health Economics*, 6: 217–227.

Chancellor, J. V., Hill, A. M., Sabin, C. A., Simpson, K. N. and Youle, M. (1997) 'Modelling the cost effectiveness of lamivudine/zidovudine combination therapy in HIV infection', *PharmacoEconomics*, 12: 54–66.

Commonwealth Department of Health, H. a. C. S. (1992) *Guidelines for the pharmaceutical industry on preparation of submissions to the Pharmaceutical Benefits Advisory Committee.* Canberra, APGS.

Coyle, D., Davies, L. and Drummond, M. (1998) 'Trials and tribulations – emerging issues in designing economic evaluations alongside clinical trials', *International Journal of Technology Assessment in Health Care*, 14: 135–144.

Culyer, A. J. (1989) 'The normative economics of health care finance and provision', *Oxford Review of Economic Policy*, 5: 34–58.

Diener, A., O'Brien, B. and Gafni, A. (1998) 'Health care contingent valuation studies: a review and classification of the literature', *Health Economics*, 7: 313–326.

Drummond, M. F. and Davies, L. (1991) 'Economic analysis alongside clinical trials', *International Journal of Technology Assessment in Health Care*, 7: 561–573.

Drummond, M. F., Sculpher, M. J., Torrance, G. W., O'Brien, B. and Stoddart, G. L. (2005) *Methods for the economic evaluation of health care programmes.* Oxford, Oxford University Press.

Freemantle, N. and Drummond, M. (1997) 'Should clinical trials with concurrent economic analyses be blinded', *Journal of the American Medical Association*, 277: 63–64.

Gafni, A. (1991) 'Willingness to pay as a measure of benefits', *Medical Care*, 29: 1246–1252.

Garber, A. M. and Phelps, C. E. (1997) 'Economic foundations of cost-effectiveness analysis'. 16: 1–31.

Gold, M. R., Siegel, J. E., Russell, L. B. and Weinstein, M. C. (1996) *Cost-effectiveness in health and medicine.* New York, Oxford University Press.

Gottlieb, J. E. and Pauker, S. G. (1981) 'Whether or not to administer amphotericin to an immunosuppressed patient with hematologic malignancy and undiagnosed fever', *Medical Decision Making*, 1: 569–587.

Hjelmgren, J., Berggren, F. and Andersson, F. (2001) 'Health economic guidelines – similarities, differences and some implications', *Value in Health*, 4: 225–250.

Hoffmann, C., Graf von der Schulenburg, J.-M. and on behalf of the EUROMET group (2000) 'The influence of economic evaluation studies on decision making: a European survey', *Health Policy*, 52: 179–192.

Hunink, M., Glaziou, P., Siegel, J., Weeks, J., Pliskin, J., Elstein, A., *et al.* (2001) *Decision making in health and medicine. Integrating evidence and values.* Cambridge, Cambridge University Press.

Johanesson, P. O. (1995) *Evaluating health risks.* Cambridge University Press, Cambridge.

Johannesson, M. and Weinstein, S. (1993) 'On the decision rules of cost-effectiveness analysis', *Journal of Health Economics*, 12: 459–467.

Loomes, G. and McKenzie, L. (1989) 'The use of QALYs in health care decision making', *Social Science and Medicine*, 28: 299–308.

McNeil, B. J., Hessel, S. J., Branch, W. T. and Bjork, L. (1976) 'Measures of Clinical Efficiency. III. The Value of the lung scan in the evaluation of young patients with pleuritic chest pain', *Journal of Nuclear Medicine*, 17(3): 163–169.

Meltzer, D. (1997) 'Accounting for future costs in medical cost-effectiveness analysis', *Journal of Health Economics*, 16: 33–64.

Ministry of Health (1994) *Ontario guidelines for economic analysis of pharmaceutical products.* Ontario, Ministry of Health.

National Institute for Clinical Excellence (NICE) (2004*a*) *Guide to technology appraisal process.* London, NICE.

National Institute for Clinical Excellence (NICE) (2004*b*) *Guide to the methods of technology appraisal.* London, NICE.

Ng, Y. K. (1983) *Welfare economics: introduction and development of basic concepts.* London, Macmillan.

Patrick, D. L. and Erickson, P. (1993) *Health status and health policy. Allocating resources to health care.* New York, Oxford University Press.

Pauly, M. V. (1995) 'Valuing health benefits in monetary terms' in F. A. Sloan (ed.) *Valuing health care: costs, benefits and effectiveness of pharmaceuticals and other medical technologies.* Cambridge, Cambridge University Press.

Pliskin, J. S., Shepard, D. S. and Weinstein, M. C. (1980) 'Utility functions for life years and health status', *Operations Research*, 28(1): 206–224.

Pritchard, C. (1998) 'Trends in economic evaluation'. OHE Briefing 36. London, Office of Health Economics.

Raiffa, H. (1968) *Decision analysis: introductory lectures on choices under uncertainty.* Reading, MA, Addison-Wesley.

Raiffa, H. and Schlaifer, R. (1959) *Probability and statistics for business decisions.* New York, McGraw-Hill.

Sackett, D. L., Rosenberg, W. M. C., Gray, J. A. M., Haynes, R. B. and Richardson, W. S. (1996) 'Evidence-based medicine: what it is and what it isn't', *British Medical Journal*, 312: 71–72.

Schoenbaum, S. C., McNeil, B. J. and Kavet, J. (1976) 'The swine-influenza decision', *New England Journal of Medicine*, 295: 759–765.

Schulman, K. A., Kinosian, B., Jacobson, T. A., Glick H., Willian M. K., Koffer H. and Eisenberg J. M. (1990) 'Reducing high blood cholesterol level with drugs: cost-effectiveness of pharmacologic management', *Journal of the American Medical Association*, 264: 3025–3033.

Sculpher, M. J. and Buxton, M. J. (1993) 'The episode-free day as a composite measure of effectiveness', *PharmacoEconomics*, 4: 345–352.

Sculpher, M., Claxton, K. and Akehurst, R. (2005) 'It's just evaluation for decision making: recent developments in, and challenges for, cost-effectiveness research' in P. C. Smith, L. Ginnelly and M. Sculpher (eds) *Health policy and economics. opportunities and challenges.* Maidenhead, Open University Press.

Sheldon, T. A. (1996) 'Problems of using modelling in the economic evaluation of health care', *Health Economics*, 5: 1–11.

Sloan, F. E. (1995) *Valuing health care: costs, benefits and effectiveness of pharmaceuticals and other medical technologies.* Cambridge, Cambridge University Press.

Sox, H. C., Blatt, M. A., Higgins, M. C. and Marton, K. I. (1988) *Medical decision making.* Stoneham, MA, Butterworths.

Stinnett, A. A. and Paltiel, A. D. (1996) 'Mathematical programming for the efficient allocation of health care resources', *Journal of Health Economics*, 15: 641–653.

Sugden, R. and Williams, A. H. (1979) *The principles of practical cost-benefit analysis.* Oxford, Oxford University Press.

Sutton, A. J. and Abrams, K. R. (2001) 'Bayesian methods in meta-analysis and evidence synthesis', *Statistical methods in medical research*, 10: 277–303.

Thompson, S. G. and Barber, J. A. (2000) 'How should cost data in pragmatic randomised trials be analysed?', *British Medical Journal*, 320: 1197–1200.

Torrance, G. W. (1986) 'Measurement of health state utilities for economic appraisal – a review', *Journal of Health Economics*, 5: 1–30.

Torrance, G. W. and Feeny, D. (1989) 'Utilities and quality-adjusted life years', *International Journal of Technology Assessment in Health Care*, 5: 559–575.

Weinstein, M. C. and Fineberg, H. V. (1980) *Clinical decision analysis.* Philadelphia, PA, WB Saunders Company.

Weinstein, M. C. and Manning, W. G. (1997) 'Theoretical issues in cost-effectiveness analysis', *Journal of Health Economics*, 16: 121–128.

Chapter 2

Key aspects of decision modelling for economic evaluation

This chapter considers the basic elements of decision modelling for economic evaluation. It considers the key stages in developing a decision analytic model and describes the cohort model, the main type of decision model used in the field. The decision tree and Markov model are described in detail and examples provided of their use in economic evaluation.

2.1. The stages of developing a decision model

It is possible to identify a series of stages in developing a decision model for economic evaluation. In part, this will involve some general choices concerning the nature of the evaluation. This will include the measure of effect and the time horizon, but also the perspective of the analysis; that is, whose costs and effects we are interested in? Below is a list of the stages in the development process which relate specifically to the decision modelling.

2.1.1. Specifying the decision problem

This involves clearly identifying the question to be addressed in the analysis. This requires a definition of the recipient population and subpopulations. This will typically be the relevant patients, but may include nonpatients (e.g. in the case of screening and prevention programmes). This requires specific details about the characteristics of individuals, but should also include information about the locations (e.g. the UK NHS) and setting (e.g. secondary care) in which the options are being delivered. The specific options being evaluated also need to be detailed. These will usually be programmes or interventions, but could include sequences of treatments with particular starting and stopping rules.

Part of the definition of the decision problem relates to which institution(s) is/are (assumed to be) making the relevant decision. In some cases this will be explicitly stated – for example, in the case of a submission to a reimbursement agency – but it will often have to be implied by the characteristics of the evaluation, such as the sources of data used.

2.1.2. Defining the boundaries of the model

All models are simplifications of reality and it will never be possible for a model to include all the possible ramifications of the particular option being considered. Choices need to be taken, therefore, about which of the possible consequences of the options under evaluation will be formally modelled. For example, should the possible implications of antibiotic resistance be assessed in all economic evaluations of interventions for infectious diseases? Another example relates to whether or not to include changes in disease transmission resulting from screening programmes for HIV. It has been shown that including reductions in the horizontal transmission of HIV in such models has a marked impact on the cost-effectiveness of screening (Sanders *et al.* 2005).

2.1.3. Structuring a decision model

Given a stated decision problem and set of model boundaries, choices have to be made about how to structure the possible consequences of the options being evaluated. In part, this will be based on the nature of the interventions themselves. For example, for an economic evaluation of alternative diagnostic strategies for urinary tract infection in children, it was necessary to use a complex decision tree to reflect the prior probability (prevalence) and diagnostic accuracy (sensitivity and specificity) of the various single and sequential screening tests (Downs 1999). In part, model structure will reflect what is known about the natural history of a particular condition and the impact of the options on that process; for example, the future risks faced by patients surviving a myocardial infarction and the impact of options for secondary prevention on those risks.

As a general approach to structuring a decision model, there is value in having some sort of underlying biological or clinical process driving the model. Examples of the former include the use of CD4 counts or viral load in HIV models (Sanders *et al.* 2005). The latter approach is more common and examples include the use of the Kurtzke Expanded Disability Status Scale in multiple sclerosis (Chilcott *et al.* 2003), the Mini Mental State Examination in Alzheimer's disease (Neumann *et al.* 1999) and clinical events, such as myocardial infarction and revascularization in coronary heart disease (Palmer *et al.* 2005). The cost-effectiveness of the relevant interventions can then be assessed by attaching health-related quality-of-life weights and costs to states or pathways defined in this way. The advantage of using these biologically- or clinically-defined states is that they should be well-understood. In particular, there should be good evidence about the natural history of a disease in terms of these definitions. This is particularly important when modelling a baseline (e.g. disease progression without treatment) and in extrapolating beyond the data from randomized trials.

There are no general rules about appropriate model structure in a given situation. However, some of the features of a disease/technology that are likely to influence choices about structure include:

- Whether the disease is acute or chronic and, if the latter, the number of possible health-related events which could occur over time.

- Whether the risks of events change over time or can reasonably be assumed to be constant.

- Whether the effectiveness of the intervention(s) (relative to some usual care baseline) can be assumed constant over time or time-limited in some way.

- If and when treatment is stopped, the appropriate assumptions about the future profile of those changes in health that were achieved during treatment. For example, would there be some sort of 'rebound' effect or would the gains, relative to a comparator group, be maintained over time (Drummond *et al.* 2005).

- Whether the probability of health-related events over time is dependent on what has happened to 'a patient' in the past.

2.1.4. **Identifying and synthesizing evidence**

The process of populating a model involves bringing together all relevant evidence, given a selected structure, and synthesizing it appropriately in terms of input parameters in the model. Consistent with the general principles of evidence-based medicine (Sackett *et al.* 1996), there needs to be a systematic approach to identifying relevant evidence. Evidence synthesis is a key area of clinical evaluation in its own right (Sutton *et al.* 2000) which is of importance outside the requirements of economic evaluation. However, the requirements of decision analytic models for economic evaluation have placed some important demands on the methods of evidence synthesis. These include:

- The need to estimate the effectiveness of interventions despite the absence of head-to-head randomized trials. This involves the use of indirect and mixed treatment comparisons to create a network of evidence between trials.

- The need to obtain probabilities of clinical events for models over a standardized period of follow-up despite the fact that clinical reports present these over varying follow-up times.

- The need for estimates of treatment effectiveness in terms of a common endpoint although trials report various measures.
- The need to assess heterogeneity in measures between different types of patients. Ideally this would be undertaken using individual patient data, but metaregression can be used with summary data in some situations.

These issues in evidence synthesis are being tackled by statisticians, often within a Bayesian framework (Sutton and Abrams 2001; Ades 2003; Spiegelhalter *et al.* 2004), and these are increasingly being used in decision models for economic evaluation (Ades *et al.* 2006). An important area of methodological research in the field relates to incorporating evidence synthesis and decision modelling into the same analytic framework – 'comprehensive decision modelling' (Parmigiani 2002; Cooper *et al.* 2004). This has the advantage of facilitating a fuller expression of the uncertainty in the evidence base in the economic evaluation.

2.1.5. Dealing with uncertainty and heterogeneity

Uncertainty and heterogeneity exist in all economic evaluations. This is an area of economic evaluation methodology that has developed rapidly in recent years (Briggs 2001), and its implications for decision modelling represent an important element of this book. Chapters 4 and 5 provide more detail about appropriate methods to handle uncertainty and heterogeneity. Box 2.1 summarizes the key concepts, and these are further developed in Chapter 4.

2.1.6. Assessing the value of additional research

The purpose of evaluative research, such as randomized control trials, is to reduce uncertainty in decision making by measuring one or more parameters (which may be specific to particular subgroups) with greater precision. This is generally true in clinical research, but also in assessing cost-effectiveness. Given limited resources, it is just as appropriate to use decision analytic models to assess the value for money of additional research projects as to assess alternative approaches to patient management. In quantifying the decision uncertainty associated with a particular comparison, decision models can provide a framework within which it is possible to begin an assessment of the cost-effectiveness of additional research. This can be undertaken informally using simple sensitivity analysis by assessing the extent to which a model's conclusions are sensitive to the uncertainty in one (or a small number)

Box 2.1. Key concept in understanding uncertainty and heterogeneity in decision models for cost-effectiveness analysis

Variability: Individual patients will inevitably differ from one another in terms, for example, of the clinical events that they experience and the associated health-related quality of life. This variability cannot be reduced through the collection of additional data.

Parameter uncertainty: The precision with which an input parameter is estimated (e.g. the probability of an event, a mean cost or a mean utility). The imprecision is a result of the fact that input parameters are estimated for *populations* on the basis of limited available information. Hence uncertainty can, in principle, be reduced through the acquisition of additional evidence.

Decision uncertainty: The joint implications of parameter uncertainty in a model result in a distribution of possible cost-effectiveness relating to the options under comparison. There is a strong normative argument for basing decisions, given available evidence, on the expectation of this distribution. But the distribution can be used to indicate the probability that the correct decision has been taken.

Heterogeneity: Heterogeneity relates to the extent to which it is possible to explain a proportion of the interpatient variability in a particular measurement on the basis of one or more patient characteristics. For example, a particular clinical event may be more likely in men and in individuals aged over 60 years. It will then be possible to estimate input parameters (and cost-effectiveness and decision uncertainty) conditional on a patient's characteristics (subgroup estimates), although uncertainty in those parameters will remain.

of parameters. Formal value-of-information methods are considered fully in Chapters 6 and 7. These methods have the strength of reflecting the joint uncertainty in all parameters. They also assess the extent to which reduction in uncertainty through additional research would result in a change in decision about the use of a technology and, if there is a change, its value in terms of improved health and/or reduced costs.

Each of these stages is crucial to the development of a decision model that is fit for the purpose of informing real policy decisions.

2.2. **Some introductory concepts in decision analysis**

Decision analysis is based on some key 'building blocks' which are common to all models. These are covered more fully in introductory texts (Weinstein and Fineberg 1980; Hunink *et al.* 2001; Drummond *et al.* 2005), and are only summarized here.

2.2.1. **Probabilities**

In decision analysis, a probability is taken as a number indicating the likelihood of an event taking place in the future. As such, decision analysis shares the same perspective as Bayesian statistics (O'Hagan and Luce 2003). This concept of probability can be generalized to represent a strength of belief which, for a given individual, is based on their previous knowledge and experience. This more 'subjective' conceptualization of probabilities is consistent with the philosophy of decision analysis, which recognizes that decisions cannot be avoided just because data are unavailable to inform them, and 'expert judgement' will frequently be necessary.

Specific probability concepts frequently used in decision analysis are:

- *Joint probability.* The probability of two events occurring concomitantly. In terms of notation, the joint probability of events A and B occurring is P(A and B).

- *Conditional probability.* The probability of an event A given that an event B is known to have occurred. The notation is P(A|B).

- *Independence.* Events A and B are independent if the probability of event A, P(A), is the same as the probability of P(A|B). When the events are independent P(A and B) = P(A) × P(B).

- Joint and conditional probabilities are related in the following equation: P(A and B) = P(A|B) × P(B). Sometimes information is available on the joint probability, and the above expression can be manipulated to 'condition out' the probabilities.

2.2.2. **Expected values**

Central to the decision analytic approach to identifying a 'preferred' option from those being compared under conditions of uncertainty is the concept of expected value. If the options under comparison relate to alternative treatments for a given patient (or an apparently homogeneous group of patients), then the structure of the decision model will reflect the variability between patients in the events that may occur with each of the treatments. The probabilities will show the likelihood of those events for a given patient. On this basis, the model will indicate a number of mutually exclusive 'prognoses' for a given patient and option (more generally, these are alternative 'states of the world' that could possibly occur with a given option). Depending on the type of model, these prognoses may be characterized, for example, as alternative pathways or sequences of states. For a given option, the likelihood of each possible prognosis can be quantified in terms of a probability, and their implications in terms of cost and/or some measure of outcome. The calculation of an expected value is shown in Box 2.2 using the example of costs. It is derived by adding together the cost of each of the possible prognoses weighted by the probability of it occurring. This is analogous to a sample mean calculated on the basis of patient-level data.

2.2.3. Payoffs

As described in the previous section, each possible 'prognosis' or 'state of the world' can be given some sort of cost or outcome. These can be termed 'payoffs', and expected values of these measures are calculated. The origins of

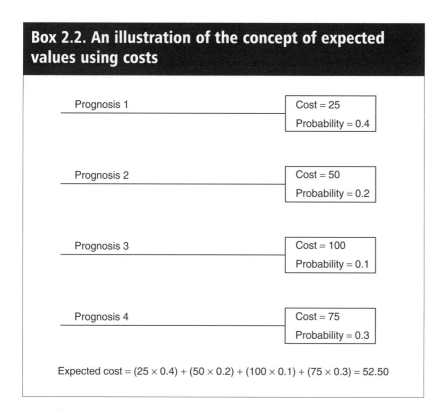

Box 2.2. An illustration of the concept of expected values using costs

Prognosis 1 — Cost = 25, Probability = 0.4

Prognosis 2 — Cost = 50, Probability = 0.2

Prognosis 3 — Cost = 100, Probability = 0.1

Prognosis 4 — Cost = 75, Probability = 0.3

Expected cost = (25 × 0.4) + (50 × 0.2) + (100 × 0.1) + (75 × 0.3) = 52.50

decision analysis are closely tied to those of expected utility theory (Raiffa 1968), so the standard payoff would have been a 'utility' as defined by von Neumann-Morgenstern (von Neumann and Morgenstern 1944). In practice, this would equate to a utility based on the standard gamble method of preference elicitation (Torrance 1986). As used for economic evaluation in health care, the payoffs in decision models have been more broadly defined. Costs would typically be one form of payoff but, on the effects side, a range of outcomes may be defined depending on the type of study (see Chapter 1). Increasingly, quality-adjusted life-years would be one of the payoffs in a decision model for cost-effectiveness analysis, which may or may not be based on utilities elicited using the standard gamble.

The principle of identifying a preferred option on the basis of a decision analytic model is on the basis of expected values. When payoffs are defined in terms of 'von Neumann-Morgenstern utilities', this would equate with a preferred option having the highest expected utility; this is consistent with expected utility theory as a normative framework for decision making under uncertainty. Although a wider set of payoffs are used in decision models for economic evaluation, the focus on expected values as a basis for decision making remains. This follows the normative theory presented by Arrow and Lind (1970) arguing that public resource allocation decisions should exhibit risk neutrality. For example, in cost-effectiveness analysis, the common incremental cost-effectiveness ratio would be based on the differences between options in terms of their expected costs and expected effects. However, the uncertainty around expected values is also important for establishing the value and design of future research, and this should also be quantified as part of a decision analytic model. The methods for quantifying and presenting uncertainty in models are described in Chapters 4 and 5, respectively; and the uses of information on uncertainty for research prioritization are considered in Chapters 6 and 7.

2.3. **Cohort models**

The overall purpose of a model structure is to characterize the consequences of alternative options in a way that is appropriate for the stated decision problem and the boundaries of the model. The structure should also be consistent with the key features of the economic evaluation, such as the perspective, time horizon and measure of outcome. There are several mathematical approaches to decision modelling from which the analyst can choose. One important consideration is whether the model should seek to characterize the experience of the 'average' patient from a population sharing the same characteristics, or should explicitly consider the individual patient and allow for variability between patients. As described previously, the focus of economic evaluation is on expected costs and effects, and uncertainty in those expected values. This has resulted in most decision models focusing on the average patient experience – these are referred to as cohort models. In certain circumstances, a more appropriate way of estimating expected values may be to move away from the cohort model, to models focused on characterizing variability between patients. These 'micro simulation' models are discussed in Chapter 3, but the focus of the remainder of this chapter is on cohort models.

The two most common forms of cohort model used in decision analysis for economic evaluation are the decision tree and the Markov model. These are considered below.

2.3.1. **The decision tree**

The decision tree is probably the simplest form of decision model. Box 2.3 provides a brief revision of the key concepts using a simple example from the management of migraine (Evans *et al.* 1997); the decision tree has been described in more detail elsewhere (Hunink *et al.* 2001; Drummond *et al.* 2005). The key features of a decision tree approach are:

- A square decision node – typically at the start of a tree – indicates a decision point between alternative options.

- A circular chance node shows a point where two or more alternative events for a patient are possible; these are shown as branches coming out of the node. For an individual patient, which event they experience is uncertain.

- Pathways are mutually exclusive sequences of events and are the routes through the tree.

- Probabilities show the likelihood of a particular event occurring at a chance node (or the proportion of a cohort of apparently homogeneous patients expected to experience the event). Moving left to right, the first probabilities in the tree show the probability of an event. Subsequent probabilities are conditional; that is, the probability of an event given that an earlier event has or has not occurred. Multiplying probabilities along pathways estimates the pathway probability which is a joint probability (as discussed previously).

Expected costs and outcomes (utilities in Box 2.3) are based on the principles in Box 2.2. Expected values are based on the summation of the pathway values weighted by the pathway probabilities.

A somewhat more complicated decision tree model comes from a cost-effectiveness analysis of alternative pharmaceutical therapies for

Box 2.3. Example of a decision tree based on Evans *et al.* (1997)

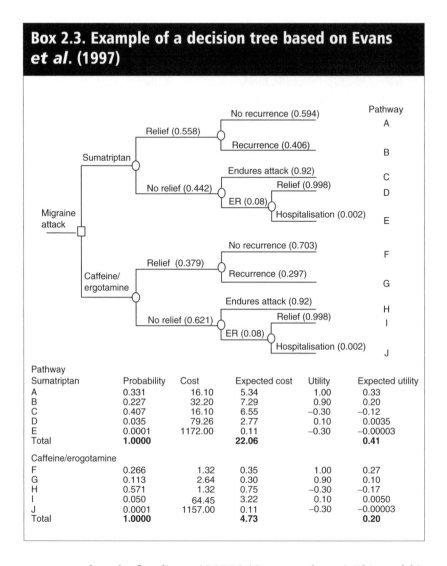

Pathway Sumatriptan	Probability	Cost	Expected cost	Utility	Expected utility
A	0.331	16.10	5.34	1.00	0.33
B	0.227	32.20	7.29	0.90	0.20
C	0.407	16.10	6.55	−0.30	−0.12
D	0.035	79.26	2.77	0.10	0.0035
E	0.0001	1172.00	0.11	−0.30	−0.00003
Total	**1.0000**		**22.06**		**0.41**
Caffeine/erogotamine					
F	0.266	1.32	0.35	1.00	0.27
G	0.113	2.64	0.30	0.90	0.10
H	0.571	1.32	0.75	−0.30	−0.17
I	0.050	64.45	3.22	0.10	0.0050
J	0.0001	1157.00	0.11	−0.30	−0.00003
Total	**1.0000**		**4.73**		**0.20**

gastro-oesophageal reflux disease (GORD) (Goeree *et al.* 1999). This model is described in some detail here, both to ensure an understanding of the decision tree, and to set up the case study used in Chapter 5 where the same model is used to demonstrate the appropriate analysis of a probabilistic model.

As shown in Fig. 2.1, six treatment options are considered in the form of strategies, as they define sequences of treatments rather than individual therapies:

◆ *A: Intermittent proton-pump inhibitor (PPI)*. Patients would be given PPI and, if this heals the GORD, they would taken off therapy. If they experience

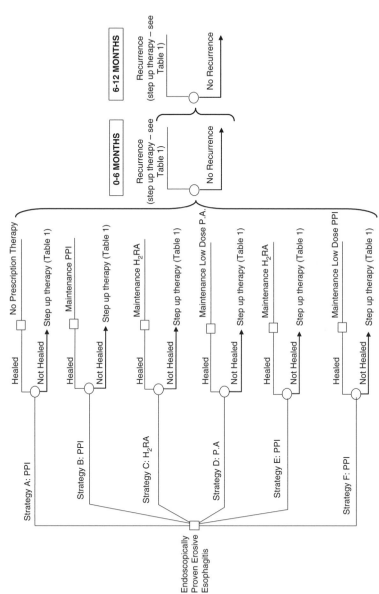

Fig. 2.1 Decision tree used to evaluate six treatment strategies for gastro-oesophageal reflux disease (adapted from Goeree *et al.* (1999)). PPP, proton pump inhibitor; H₂RA: H₂ receptor antagonists; PA: prokinetic agent. Table 1 refers to the table from the original article.

a recurrence of the condition, they would be returned to the PPI regimen. If patients fail to heal with their initial dose of PPI, the dose of the therapy would be doubled (DD PPI) and, once healed, patients would be maintained on standard dose PPI. If the GORD recurs, they would be given DD PPI.

- B: *Maintenance PPI*. Patients would initially be treated with PPI and, once healed, they would be maintained on PPI. If they fail to heal with their initial dose, or if the GORD recurs subsequent to healing, they would be given DD PPI.

- C: *Maintenance H_2 receptor antagonists (H_2RA)*. Patients are initially treated with H_2RA and, if they heal, they are maintained on that drug. If their GORD subsequently recurs, they are placed on double-dose H_2RA (DD H_2RA). If patients fail to heal on the initial dose, they are given PPI and, if they then heal, are maintained with H_2RA. If the GORD subsequently recurs, they are given PPI to heal. If patients fail to heal initially with PPI, they are moved to DD PPI and, if they then heal, are maintained with PPI. If the GORD subsequently recurs on maintenance PPI, they are given DD PPI to heal.

- D: *Step-down maintenance prokinetic agent (PA)*. Patients would be given PA for initial healing and, if this is successful, maintained on low dose (LD) PA; if their GORD subsequently recurs, they would be put on PA to heal again. If patients fail their initial healing dose of PA, they would be moved to PPI to heal and, if successful, maintained on LD PA. If their GORD subsequently recurs, they would be treated with PPI for healing. If patients fail their initial healing dose of PPI, they would be moved to DD PPI and, if successful, maintained on PPI. If the GORD subsequently recurs, they would receive DD PPI to heal.

- E: *Step-down maintenance H_2RA*. Patients would initially receive PPI to heal and, if this is successful, they would be maintained on H_2RA. If they subsequently recur, they would be given PPI to heal. Patients who initially fail on PPI would be given DD PPI and, if this heals the GORD, they would be maintained on PPI. If their GORD subsequently recurs, healing would be attempted with DD PPI.

- F: *Step-down maintenance PPI*. Patients would initially be treated with PPI and, if this heals the GORD, would move to LD PPI. In the case of a subsequent recurrence, patients would be given PPI to heal. Patients who fail on their initial dose of PPI would be given DD PPI and, if successful, maintained on PPI. If their GORD recurs, they would be given DD PPI to heal.

The structure of the decision tree used in the study is shown in Fig. 2.1. For each strategy, the initial pathway shows whether their GORD initially heals and, if so, it indicates the maintenance therapy a patient will move to. If they do not heal, they move to step up therapy as defined for each of the five strategies. The figure shows that, for each pathway on the tree, there is a probability of GORD recurrence during two periods: 0–6 months and 6–12 months. Should this happen, step-up therapy is used as defined above. It should be noted that the tree contains decision nodes to the right of chance nodes. However, this indicates a treatment decision defined by the strategies rather than a point in the tree where alternative courses of action are being compared.

To populate the model, the authors undertook a meta-analysis of randomized trials to estimate, for each drug, the proportion of patients healed at different time points. They also used available trial data to calculate the proportions of patients who recur with GORD over the two time periods. Routine evidence sources and clinical opinion were used to estimate the cost of therapies and of recurrence.

The decision tree was evaluated over a time horizon of 12 months. Costs were considered from the perspective of the health system and outcomes were expressed in terms of the expected number of weeks (out of 52) during which a patient was free of GORD. Table 2.1 shows the base-case results of the analysis. For each strategy over 1 year, it shows the expected costs and time with (and without) GORD symptoms. The table shows the options that are dominated or subject to extended dominance (Johannesson and Weinstein 1993), and the incremental cost per week of GORD symptoms avoided are shown for the remaining options. Figure 2.2 shows the base-case cost-effectiveness results on the cost-effectiveness plane (Black 1990; Johannesson and Weinstein 1993). It shows that Option D is dominated as it is more costly and less effective than Options C, A and E. It also shows that Option F is subject to extended dominance. That is, it lies to the left of the efficiency frontier defined by non-dominated options. This means that it would be possible to give a proportion of patients Option E and a proportion Option B and the combined costs and effects of this mixed option would dominate Option F (see the discussion of cost-effectiveness decision rules in Chapter 1).

2.3.2. Markov models

The advantages of Markov models

Although various aspects of the GORD case study, such as the choice of outcome measure, can be criticized, the study provides a good example of a cost-effectiveness model based around a decision tree structure. Some of the

Table 2.1 Base-case results from the gastro-oesophageal reflux disease case study (Goeree et al. 1999)

Strategy	Expected 1-year cost per patient $	Expected weeks with (without) GORD per patient in 1 year	Incremental costs (DC) $	Incremental effects (DE) GORD weeks averted	DC/DE ($/GORD week averted)
C: Maintenance H₂RA	657	10.41 (41.59)	–	–	–
A: Intermittent PPI	678	7.78 (44.22)	21	2.63	8
E: Step-down maintenance H₂RA	748	6.17 (45.83)	70*	1.61*	44*
B: Maintenance PPI	1093	4.82 (47.18)	345†	1.35†	256†
D: Step-down maintenance PA	805	12.60 (39.40)			Dominated by A,C,E
F: Step-down maintenance PPI	955	5.54 (46.46)			Dominated by extended dominance

* Relative to strategy A

† Relative to strategy E

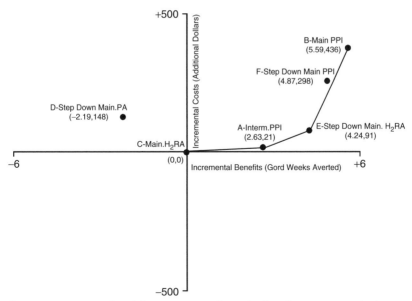

Fig. 2.2 Base-case results of the gastro-oesophageal reflux disease case study shown on the cost-effectiveness plane (taken from Goeree *et al.* (1999)). The line joining Strategies C, A, E and B is the 'efficiency frontier'.

potential limitations of the decision tree are also evident in the case study. The first is that the elapse of time is not explicit in decision trees. GORD relapse between 0 and 6 months and between 6 and 12 months has to be separately built into the model as no element of the structure explicitly relates to failure rate over time.

A second limitation of decision trees made evident in the GORD example is the speed with which the tree format can become unwieldy. In the GORD case study, only three consequences of interventions are directly modelled: initial healing, relapse between 0 and 6 months and relapse between 6 and 12 months. GORD is a chronic condition and it can be argued that for this analysis, a lifetime time horizon may have been more appropriate than one of 12 months. If a longer time horizon had been adopted, several further features of the model structure would have been necessary. The first is the need to reflect the continuing risk of GORD recurrence (and hence the need for step-up therapy) over time. The second is the requirement to allow for the competing risk of death as the cohort ages. The third is the consideration of other clinical developments, such as the possible occurrence of oesophageal cancer in patients experiencing recurrent GORD over a period of years. This pattern of recurring-remitting disease over a period of many years and of competing clinical risks is characteristic of many chronic diseases such as diabetes, ischaemic heart disease and some forms of cancer. In such situations, the need to reflect a large number of possible consequences over time would result in the decision tree becoming very 'bushy' and, therefore, difficult to program and to present. As such, a Markov framework was used to further develop the GORD model described above (Goeree *et al.* 2002).

The Markov model is a commonly used approach in decision analysis to handle the added complexity of modelling options with a multiplicity of possible consequences. Such models have been used in the evaluation of screening programmes (Sanders *et al.* 2005), diagnostic technologies (Kuntz *et al.* 1999) and therapeutic interventions (Sculpher *et al.* 1996). The added flexibility of the Markov model relates to the fact that it is structured around mutually exclusive disease states, representing the possible consequences of the options under evaluation. Instead of possible consequences over time being modelled as a large number of possible pathways as in a decision tree, a more complex prognosis is reflected as a set of possible transitions between the disease states over a series of discrete time periods (cycles). Costs and effects are typically incorporated into these models as a mean value per state per cycle, and expected values are calculated by adding the costs and outcomes across the states and weighting according to the time the patient is expected to be in each state.

A case study in HIV

The details of the Markov model can be illustrated using a case study. This is a cost-effectiveness analysis of zidovudine monotherapy compared with zidovudine plus lamivudine (combination) therapy in patients with HIV infection (Chancellor *et al.* 1997). This example has been used for didactic purposes before (Drummond *et al.* 2005), but is further developed here, and in Chapter 4 for purposes of probabilistic analysis.

The structure of the Markov model is shown in Fig. 2.3. This model characterizes a patient's prognosis in terms of four states. Two of these are based on CD4 count: 200–500 cells/mm^3 (the least severe disease state – State A) and less than 200 cells/mm^3 (State B). The third state is AIDS (State C) and the final state is death (State D). The arrows on the Markov diagram indicate the transitions patients can make in the model. The key structural assumption in this early HIV model (now clinically doubtful, at least in developed countries) is that patients can only remain in the same state or progress; it is not feasible for them to move back to a less severe state. More recent models have allowed patients to move back from an AIDS state to non-AIDS states and, through therapy, to experience an increase in CD4 count. These models have also

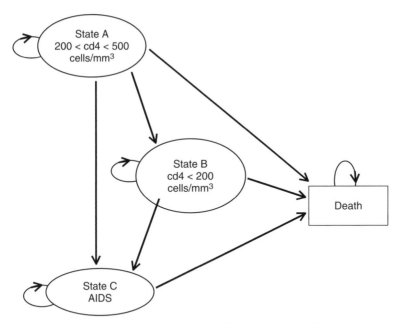

Fig. 2.3 The structure of the Markov model used in the case study (Chancellor *et al.* 1997).

allowed for the fact that prognosis for these patients is now understood in terms of viral load as well as CD4 count (Sanders *et al.* 2005).

The transition probabilities governing the direction and speed of transitions between disease states in the model are shown in Table 2.2 where a cycle is taken as 1 year. For monotherapy, these 'baseline' (i.e. control group) probabilities are taken from a longitudinal cohort study where data were collected prior to any use of combination therapy. The zeros indicate that backwards transitions are assumed not to be feasible. The transition probabilities for combination therapy were based on an adjustment to the baseline values according to the treatment effect of combination therapy relative to monotherapy. This treatment effect took the form of a relative risk (0.509) which was derived from a meta-analysis of trials. Although the treatment effect in the trials was something rather different, it was assumed that the relative risk worked to reduce the transition probabilities from one state to any worse state. The calculation of these revised (combination) transition probabilities is shown in Table 2.2. Any probability relating to the movement to a worse state is multiplied by 0.509, and the probability of remaining in a state is correspondingly increased. The separation of baseline probabilities from a relative

Table 2.2 Transition probabilities and costs for the HIV Markov model used in the case study (Chancellor *et al*. 1997)

State at start of cycle	State at end of cycle			
1. Annual transition probabilities				
(a) Monotherapy				
	State A	State B	State C	State D
State A	0.721	0.202	0.067	0.010
State B	0.000	0.581	0.407	0.012
State C	0.000	0.000	0.750	0.250
State D	0.000	0.000	0.000	0.000
(b) Combination therapy				
	State A	State B	State C	State D
State A	0.858	0.103	0.034	0.005
	(1 − sum)	(0.202 × RR)	(0.067 × RR)	(0.010 × RR)
State B	0.000	0.787	0.207	0.006
		(1 − sum)	(0.407 × RR)	(0.012 × RR)
State C	0.000	0.000	0.873	0.127
			(1 − sum)	(0.25 × RR)
State D	0.000	0.000	0.000	1.000
2. Annual costs				
Direct medical	£1701	£1774	£6948	–
Community	£1055	£1278	£2059	–
Total	£2756	£3052	£9007	–

RR, relative risk of disease progression. Estimated as 0.509 in a meta-analysis.

The drug costs were £2278 (zidovudine) and £2086 (lamivudine).

treatment effect is a common feature of many decision models used for cost-effectiveness. One advantage of this approach relates to the important task of estimating cost-effectiveness for a particular location and population subgroup. Often it is assumed that baseline event probabilities should be as specific as possible to the location(s) and subgroup(s) of interest, but that the relative treatment effect is assumed fixed.

It can be seen that all the transition probabilities are fixed with respect to time. That is, the baseline annual probability of progressing from, for example, State A to State B is 0.202, and this is the case 1 year after start of therapy and it is also the case, for those remaining in State A, after 10 years. When these time invariant probabilities are used, this is sometimes referred to as a Markov Chain.

Table 2.2 also shows the annual costs associated with the different states. These are assumed identical for both treatment options being compared – excluding the costs of the drugs being evaluated. The drug costs were

£2278 (zidovudine) and £2086 (lamivudine). Outcomes were assessed in terms of changes in mean survival duration so no health-related quality-of-life weights (utilities) were included.

Cohort simulation

As explained previously, the calculation of expected costs and outcomes for all cohort models involves summing the costs and outcomes of all possible consequences weighted by the probability of the consequence. In the case of Markov models, this involves calculating how long patients would spend in a given disease state. This can be achieved using matrix algebra, but is more commonly undertaken using a process known as cohort simulation. This is illustrated, for the first two cycles for monotherapy, in Fig. 2.4. Exactly the same process would be used for combination therapy based on the adjusted transition probabilities in Table 2.2. This example uses a cohort size of 1000, but this number is arbitrary and, for a cohort model, the same answer will emerge for any size of starting cohort. Cohort simulation simply involves multiplying the proportion of the cohort ending in one state by the relevant transition probability to derive the proportion starting in another state. In a spreadsheet, this is achieved by setting up the formulae for one cycle and then copying down for subsequent cycles.

Calculating expected costs for a cohort model simply involves, for each cycle, adding the costs of each state weighted by the proportion in the state, and then adding across cycles. This is shown in Table 2.3 for monotherapy based on the costs shown in Table 2.2 and annual drug costs for zidovudine of £2278. The process of discounting to a present value is very straightforward in a cohort simulation and this is also shown in Table 2.3.

Table 2.4 shows the calculation of expected survival duration (life expectancy) for the monotherapy group. At its simplest, this involves adding the proportion of the living cohort for each cycle, and adding across the cycles. Of course, the units in which survival duration is estimated will depend on the cycle length. In the case study, all transitions are assumed to take place at the start of the cycle, so the simple approach to calculating life expectancy assumes those dying during a cycle do not survive for any proportion of the cycle. Strictly, an unbiased estimate of life expectancy would assume that deaths occur halfway through a cycle. It is possible, therefore, to employ a half-cycle correction as shown in the final column of Table 2.3. The half-cycle correction is shown here just for life expectancy calculation. In principle, however, it also applies to the calculation of expected costs. In the context of a cost-effectiveness analysis where the focus is on the incremental costs and outcomes of alternative options, it is unlikely that the half-cycle correction

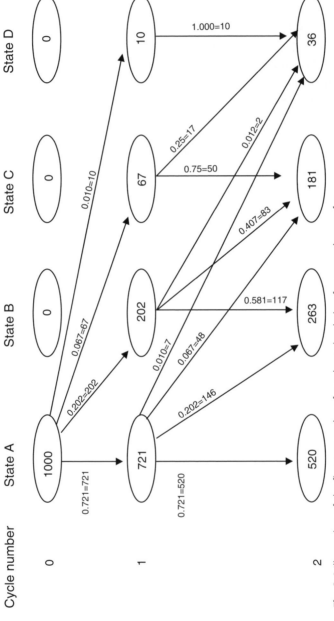

Fig. 2.4 Illustration of the first two cycles of a cohort simulation for monotherapy for the Markov model used in the case study.

Table 2.3 Calculation of expected costs for monotherapy in the case study Markov model based on the costs shown in Table 2.2, annual drug costs of £2278 and an annual discount rate of 6%

Cycle (year)	Proportion of cohort in each state				Costs (£)	
	A	B	C	D	Undiscounted	Discounted
0	1000					
1	721	202	67	10	5463*	5153†
2	520	263	181	36	6060	5393
3	376	258	277	89	6394	5368
4	271	226	338	165	6381	5055
5	195	186	364	255	6077	4541
6	141	147	361	350	5574	3929
7	102	114	341	444	4963	3301
8	73	87	309	531	4316	2708†
9	53	65	272	610	3682	2179
10	38	49	234	679	3092	1727
11	28	36	198	739	2564	1350
12	20	26	165	789	2102	1045
13	14	19	136	830	1708	801
14	10	14	111	865	1377	609
15	7	10	90	893	1103	460
16	5	8	72	915	878	346
17	4	5	57	933	695	258
18	3	4	45	948	548	192
19	2	3	36	959	431	142
20	1	2	28	968	337	105
					63 745	44 663

*{[721 × (2756 + 2278)] + [202 × (3052 + 2278)] + [67 × (9007 + 2278)] + [10 × 0]} / 1000
†5463 / [(1 + 0.06)^1]

will make a lot of difference to results unless the cycle length is long as a proportion of the model's time horizon.

Of course, the cohort simulation and calculation of expected costs and expected survival duration, shown in Fig. 2.4 and Tables 2.3 and 2.4 for the monotherapy baseline, would also need to be undertaken for combination therapy. The process would be exactly the same but would involve different transition probabilities and costs.

Table 2.4 Calculation of life expectancy over 20 cycles for monotherapy for the case study Markov model. Calculation with and without a half-cycle correction is shown

Cycle (year)	Proportion of cohort in each state				Life years	
	A	B	C	D	Die at start	Die in middle
0	1000					
1	721	202	67	10	0.990	0.995
2	520	263	181	36	0.964	0.977
3	376	258	277	89	0.911	0.937
4	271	226	338	165	0.835*	0.873
5	195	186	364	255	0.745	0.790
6	141	147	361	350	0.650	0.697
7	102	114	341	444	0.556	0.603†
8	73	87	309	531	0.469	0.513
9	53	65	272	610	0.390	0.429
10	38	49	234	679	0.321	0.355
11	28	36	198	739	0.261	0.291
12	20	26	165	789	0.211	0.236
13	14	19	136	830	0.170	0.190
14	10	14	111	865	0.135	0.152
15	7	10	90	893	0.107	0.121
16	5	8	72	915	0.085	0.096
17	4	5	57	933	0.067	0.076
18	3	4	45	948	0.052	0.059
19	2	3	36	959	0.041	0.047
20	1	2	28	968	0.032	0.036
					7.996	8.475

*(271 + 226 + 338) / 1000
†{102 + 114 + 341 + [0.5 × (444 − 350)]}/1000

The Markov assumption

Although the Markov version of a cohort model provides greater flexibility than a decision tree, it also has some important restrictions in the context of structuring complex prognoses. The restriction relates to what is known as the Markov assumption, or 'memoryless' feature of Markov models. This assumption means that once a notional patient has moved from one state to another,

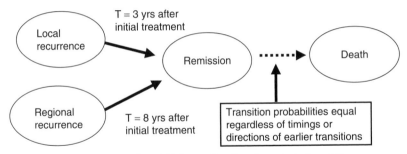

Note: T = time since initial operation (i.e. since start of model)

Fig. 2.5 Example of a simple Markov model to illustrate the Markov assumption.

the Markov model will have 'no memory' regarding where the patient has come from or the timing of that transition. This is illustrated in Fig. 2.5 using a simple Markov model to characterize prognosis following treatment for cancer. It shows that patients can have two forms of cancer recurrence: local and regional. Once treated for their recurrence, patients then move into a remission state but, once in that state, all patients are considered homogeneous regardless of where they have come from (what type of recurrence) or the timing of the recurrence after initial treatment for the cancer. The implication of this is that it is not possible to have different probabilities of future transitions (e.g. the probability of death in Fig. 2.5) according to the nature or timing of the recurrence.

In general, the Markov assumption means that it may not be straightforward to build 'history' into this type of model. That is, to model a process where future events depend on past events. This may be possible by adding additional states to the model and incorporating time dependency into transition probabilities. Both of these extensions to the Markov model are considered in Chapter 3.

2.4. **Summary**

This chapter has described some of the key concepts for the use of decision analysis for economic evaluation. The majority of cost-effectiveness studies are based on cohort modelling. This provides a flexible framework which can be programmed relatively easily (often in spreadsheets) and evaluated rapidly. However, the cohort framework can be restricting. In the case of Markov models, for example, the memoryless feature of these models can cause difficulties in modelling a complicated prognosis.

2.5. **Exercise: replicating a Markov model of HIV/AIDS**

2.5.1. **Overview**

The aim of this exercise is to get you to replicate a previously published Markov model by Chancellor and colleagues (1997). The model itself is somewhat out of date, in that it compares combination therapy (lamivudine and AZT) with monotherapy (AZT alone). Nevertheless, the model is straightforward enough to serve as a simple example that it is possible to replicate in a short period of time.

The basic structure of the model was given in Fig. 2.3, which shows that the disease process is structured as chronic, such that patients can move to successively more serious disease states, but cannot recover.

The cycle length of the model is 1 year and is evaluated over 20 years (after which more than 95 per cent of patients are expected to have died).

Use the data given below to populate the model and calculate the incremental cost-effectiveness ratio for AZT monotherapy. You should be able to replicate a figure for the ICER of £6276.

1. *Transition probabilities.* These were calculated from the counts of individuals that were observed to move between the four health states each year in a longitudinal data set from the Chelsea and Westminster Hospital in London. These counts are given in Table 2.5 and you should be able to verify that these counts give the transition probabilities presented in Table 2.2 part 1(a).

2. *State costs.* These are given in the original article separately by state for 'direct medical' and 'community care' costs and these were reproduced in Table 2.2 part 2.

3. *Costs of drugs.* The yearly cost of AZT monotheray is given as £2278 and lamivudine is given as £2086.50.

4. *Treatment effect.* A meta-analysis of four trials is reported in the paper giving a pooled relative risk of disease progression as 0.509. Note from Table 2.2 part 1(b) how this treatment effect is applied to the monotherapy transitions in the model.

Table 2.5 Counts of transition between the four model states per year

	A	B	C	D	Total
A	1251	350	116	17	1734
B	0	731	512	15	1258
C	0	0	1312	437	
D					

5. *Discounting*. The original analysis was based on discounting the costs at 6 per cent but not discounting the estimates of life years.

2.5.2. **Step-by-step guide to constructing the model**

Open the file '*Exercise 2.5 – Template*' and start at the <*Parameters*> worksheet. You will see that the cells to be completed are coloured yellow.

Using the figures from Table 2.5, complete columns C and D on the <*Parameters*> worksheet for the transition probabilities (rows 9–17). Column C should contain the number of events of interest and column D should contain the complement, such that columns C plus D should equal the appropriate row total from Table 2.5 above. Now calculate the respective transition probabilities in column B using the counts in columns C and D (the reason for structuring the spreadsheet like this will become apparent in the exercise in Chapter 4).

Enter the other information for the state costs, drug costs, treatment effect and discounting given above in the appropriate place in the template.

Having entered the input parameters of the model, the task now is to construct the Markov models for the treatment alternatives: combination and monotherapy. Note that the parameters you have just entered are in named cells, such that they can be referred to by the shortened name in column A of the <*Parameters*> worksheet.

If you move to the Markov worksheet, you will see the structure of the Markov model laid out for you for each treatment alternative. Start with the monotherapy model.

1. Generating the Markov trace

The initial concern is with generating the Markov trace, that is, showing the proportions of patients that are in any one state at any one time. This is to be entered in columns C to F representing the four model states, and G provides a check (as the sum across C to F must always equal the size of the original cohort – which is set to 1 in cell C7 such that the Markov trace represents proportions of patients).

The first step in building a Markov model is to define the transition matrix. This is a matrix that shows the probability of transition from states represented in the rows to states represented in the columns. To save you time, a copy of the transition matrix is reproduced in Table 2.6 for the monotherapy arm.

  i. Start by making sure that you understand the transition matrix. In particular, make sure you can replicate it from the information given in the diagram of the model in Fig. 2.3.

Table 2.6 Transition matrix for the monotherapy arm

Transition matrix	A	B	C	D
A	tpA2A	tpA2B	tpA2C	tpA2D
B	0	tpB2B	tpB2C	tpB2D
C	0	0	tpC2C	tpC2D
D	0	0	0	1

ii. Use the transition matrix to populate the Markov model. This will involve representing the transitions between the different states represented in columns C to F.

Hints: Start with just one row at a time (e.g. the first – row 8). Once you have this row correct you can simply copy it down to the other rows. Although it is tempting to look across the rows of the transition matrix – consider looking down the columns as this indicates, for a given state, where the people entering that state come from. Indeed, the transition matrix describes the proportion of patients in the other states in the previous cycle arriving in the given state for this cycle. For example, looking down for 'State B' we find that tpA2B patients in 'State A' last period arrive in State B this period and that tpB2B patients in 'State B' last period stay in 'State B' this period. The formula for cell D8 should therefore read: =C7*tpA2B+D7*tpB2B

iii. When you get to the dead state, do not be tempted to make this the remainder of the other cells in the row – the use of remainders in this way will mean that any errors could go unnoticed. Instead, it is good practice to complete all states as you think they should be then sum across the states to make sure the total sums to one. Do this check in column G and make sure it does!

iv. When you think you have the first row correct, copy this row down to the 19 rows below. If your check in column G is still looking good then most likely you have done it correctly.

By far the most tricky bit of building the Markov model in Excel is now complete. Now that you have the Markov trace you can calculate the cost and effects.

2. Estimating life years

In column H calculate the proportion of the cohort that is in one of the 'alive' states for each of the years in the model. In column I apply the standard discount formula[1] (although we have set this to zero in the base case). Finally, in row 29, sum the columns to give the expected life years both discounted and undiscounted.

3. Estimating costs

In column K, calculate the costs for each time period by applying the state costs, not forgetting that AZT is given for the whole time period. In column L, apply the standard rate of discount for costs. Again, in Row 29, sum the columns to give costs both undiscounted and discounted.

4. Adapting the model for combination therapy

You now need to repeat the steps above, but this time for combination therapy.

    i. Start by copying the whole monotherapy model to the corresponding combination therapy model. This will minimize repetition as tasks now relate to adjusting the model for combination treatment. (Note: remember to anchor the year (column A) in the discounting formula before copying).

    ii. Firstly, the treatment effect needs to be added in. In the original article, the relative risk parameter was applied to all transitions. The corresponding transition matrix for combination therapy is, therefore, given in Table 2.7.

    iii. Use this transition matrix to adjust the trace in rows 8 and 9 only (as the base case assumption in the originally reported model was that treatment effect was limited to 2 years).

Now add in the cost of lamivudine for these 2 years only in column V (as the drug is assumed to be given for only 2 years)

....

[1] Recall that the standard discount rate is given by $1/(1 + r)^t$ where r is the discount rate and t represents time (in years).

Table 2.7 Transition matrix for the combination therapy arm

Transition matrix	A	B	C	D
A	1-tpA2B*RR-tpA2C*RR-tpA2D*RR	tpA2B*RR	tpA2C*RR	tpA2D*RR
B	0	1-tpB2C*RR-tpB2D*RR	tpB2C*RR	tpB2D*RR
C	0	0	1-tpC2D*RR	tpC2D*RR
D	0	0	0	1

5. Cost-effectiveness estimates

The final task is simply to copy the corresponding results from the sums at the bottom of the Markov model sheet (row 29) to the *<Analysis>* worksheet (row 5) and to calculate the appropriate increments and ICER.

Congratulations, you have now replicated the Markov model. Compare your result for the ICER to that given in the solution (£6276). Is any debugging required? If it is, then you may want to compare your Markov trace and stage costs for monotherapy against those reported in Table 2.3.

References

Ades, A. E. (2003) A chain of evidence with mixed comparisons: models for multi-parameter evidence synthesis and consistency of evidence, *Statistics in Medicine*, 22: 2995–3016.

Ades, A. E., Sculpher, M. J., Sutton, A., Abrams, K., Cooper, N., Welton, N., *et al.* (2006) 'Bayesian methods for evidence synthesis in cost-effectiveness analysis', *PharmacoEconomics* 24: 1–19.

Arrow, K. J. and Lind, R. C. (1970) 'Risk and uncertainty: uncertainty and the evaluation of public investment decisions', *American Economic Review*, 60: 364–78.

Black, W. C. (1990) 'The CE plane: a graphic representation of cost-effectiveness', *Medical Decision Making*, 10: 212–214.

Briggs, A. (2001) 'Handling uncertainty in economic evaluation and presenting the results' in M. Drummond and A. J. McGuire (eds) *Economic evaluation in health care: merging theory with practice*. Oxford, Oxford University Press; pp. 172–214.

Chancellor, J. V., Hill, A. M., Sabin, C. A., Simpson, K. N. and Youle, M. (1997) 'Modelling the cost effectiveness of lamivudine/zidovudine combination therapy in HIV infection', *PharmacoEconomics*, 12: 1–13.

Chilcott, J., McCabe, C., Tappenden, P., O'Hagan, A., Cooper, N. J., Abrams, K., *et al.* (2003) 'Modelling the cost effectiveness of interferon beta and glatiramer acete in the management of multiple sclerosis', *British Medical Journal*, 326: 522.

Cooper, N. J., Sutton, A. J., Abrams, K. R., Turner, D. and Wailoo, A. (2004) 'Comprehensive decision analytical modelling in economic evaluation: A Bayesian approach', *Health Economics*, 13: 203–226.

Downs, S. (1999) 'Technical report: urinary tract infections in febrile infants and young children', *Pediatrics*, 103: 54.

Drummond, M. F., Sculpher, M. J., Torrance, G. W., O'Brien, B. and Stoddart, G. L. (2005). *Methods for the economic evaluation of health care programmes*. Oxford, Oxford University Press.

Evans, K. W., Boan, J. A., Evans, J. L. and Shuaib, A. (1997) 'Economic evaluation of oral sumatriptan compared with oral caffeine/ergotamine for migraine', *PharmacoEconomics*, 12: 565–577.

Goeree, R., O'Brien, B. J., Hunt, R., Blackhouse, G., Willan, A. and Watson, J. (1999) 'Economic evaluation of long term management strategies for erosive oesphagitis', *PharmacoEconomics*, 16: 679–697.

Goeree, R., O'Brien, B. J., Blackhouse, G., Marshall, J., Briggs, A. H. and Lad, R. (2002) 'Cost-effectiveness and cost-utility of long-term management strategies for heartburn', *Value in Health*, 5: 312–328.

Hunink, M., Glaziou, P., Siegel, J., Weeks, J., Pliskin, J., Elstein, A., *et al.* (2001) *Decision making in health and medicine. Integrating evidence and values.* Cambridge, Cambridge University Press.

Johannesson, M. and Weinstein, S. (1993) 'On the decision rules of cost-effectiveness analysis', *Journal of Health Economics,* 12: 459–467.

Kuntz, K. M., Fleishmann, K. E., Hunink, M. G. M. and Douglas, P. S. (1999) 'Cost-effectiveness of diagnostic strategies for patients with chest pain', *Annals of Internal Medicine,* 130: 709–718.

Neumann, P. J., Hermann, R. C. and Kuntz, K. M. (1999) 'Cost-effectiveness of donepezil in the treatment of mild or moderate Alzheimer's disease', *Neurology,* 52: 1138–45.

O'Hagan, A. and Luce, B. (2003) *A primer on Bayesian statistics in health economics and outcomes research.* Bethesda, MD, Medtap International.

Palmer, S., Sculpher, M., Philips, Z., Robinson, M., Ginnelly, L., Bakhai, A., *et al.* (2005) 'Management of non-ST-elevation acute coronary syndromes: how cost-effective are glycoprotein IIb/IIIa antagonists in the UK National Health Service?', *International Journal of Cardiology,* 100: 229–240.

Parmigiani, G. (2002) *Modeling in medical decision making: a Bayesian approach.* Chichester, Wiley.

Raiffa, H. (1968) *Decision analysis: introductory lectures on choices under uncertainty.* Reading, MA, Addison-Wesley.

Sackett, D. L., Rosenberg, W. M. C., Gray, J. A. M., Haynes, R. B. and Richardson, W. S. (1996) 'Evidence-based medicine: what it is and what it isn't', *British Medical Journal,* 312: 71–72.

Sanders, G. D., Bayoumi, A. M., Sundaram, V., Bilir, S. P., Neukermans, C. P. and *et al.* (2005) 'Cost-effectiveness of screening for HIV in the era of highly active antiretroviral therapy', *New England Journal of Medicine,* 352: 570–585.

Sculpher, M., Michaels, J., McKenna, M. and Minor, J. (1996) 'A cost-utility analysis of laser-assisted angioplasty for peripheral arterial occlusions', International Journal of Technology Assessment in Health Care 12: 104–125.

Spiegelhalter, D. J., Abrams, K. R. and Myles, J. P. (2004). *Bayesian approaches to clinical trials and health-care evaluation.* Chichester, Wiley.

Sutton, A. J. and Abrams, K. R. (2001) 'Bayesian methods in meta-analysis and evidence synthesis', *Statistical Methods in Medical Research,* 10: 277–303.

Sutton, A. J., Abrams, K. R., Jones, D. R., Sheldon, T. A. and Song, T. A. (2000) *Methods for meta-analysis in medical research.* Chichester, Wiley.

Torrance, G. W. (1986) 'Measurement of health state utilities for economic appraisal – a review', *Journal of Health Economics,* 5: 1–30.

von Neumann, J. and Morgenstern, O. (1944) *Theory of games and economic behavior.* New York, Princeton University Press.

Weinstein, M. C. and Fineberg, H. V. (1980) *Clinical decision analysis.* Philadelphia, PA, WB Saunders Company.

Chapter 3

Further developments in decision analytic models for economic evaluation

As a framework for economic evaluation, decision analysis needs adequately to reflect the key features of the natural history of a disease and the impact of alternative programmes and interventions. Models are, however, simplifications of reality and will always approximate these phenomena. In short, to be 'fit for purpose' for decision making, decision models need to strike a balance between realism and flexibility in terms of computation and data requirements. Chapter 2 described the two basic types of decision model that predominate in economic evaluation: the decision tree and the Markov model. These models can be used for a wide range of decision problems. In some circumstances, however, their structural assumptions are clearly at odds with the theory and/or evidence associated with a particular disease or technology. In such cases, it may be appropriate to develop the models further in one or more key respects.

This chapter considers some of the further developments that might be considered for decision models to increase the extent to which they fit with what is known about a disease or the relevant interventions. The following section describes ways in which greater 'complexity' can be added to cohort models. The next main section describes the use of patient-level simulation models in economic evaluation, and the subsequent section considers the use of dynamic models in the context of infectious diseases.

3.1. Extensions to cohort models

Cohort models are the mainstay of decision analysis for economic evaluation. This is because they can balance an adequate reflection of available knowledge and evidence regarding a disease and interventions with parsimony in terms of computation and data. For certain types of decision problem, it is important to go beyond the simple decision tree or Markov model. Here, three extensions to the simple cohort model are described: the combination of the decision tree and the cohort model; adding time-dependency; and loosening the memoryless restriction of the Markov model.

3.1.1. **Combining decision trees and Markov models**

Although they are described as distinct forms of model in Chapter 2, it would be a mistake to see Markov models and decision trees as mutually exclusive; indeed, Markov models are really just a form of recursive decision tree. For some evaluations, they can be used jointly. One form of this is when transitions between Markov states are characterized in terms of a tree – these have been called Markov cycle trees (Hollenberg 1984). A model can also be made up of multiple elements involving one or more tree and Markov model. An example of this is a cost-effectiveness analysis of glycoprotein IIb/IIIa (GPA) drugs in non-ST-elevation acute coronary syndrome (NSTACS) (Palmer *et al.* 2005). As shown in Fig. 3.1, a decision tree was used to characterize the possible short-term events following an acute episode of NSTACS under one of four strategies (three based on the use of GPAs and one 'usual care' strategy without these drugs). The short-term period was 6 months, which represented the longest period of follow-up in most of the GPA trials.

The ultimate purpose of the decision tree was to estimate, for each of the four strategies, the proportion of the patient cohort in each of three states at 6 months: dead, alive having not experienced a myocardial infarction but remaining with ischaemic heart disease (IHD), and alive having experienced a myocardial infarction. The objective of the Markov model was to estimate the expected quality-adjusted survival duration and lifetime costs for the cohort. Hence, the differences between therapies only relate to the first 6 months; the Markov model estimates long-term survival duration and costs conditional on the patient's status at 6 months, but does not differentiate between initial treatments. The Markov model allows for the fact that, over the longer term, patients will continue to be at risk of myocardial infarction. The reason for there being two myocardial infarction states in the Markov model is that evidence suggested that patients' risk of death and their costs are higher following myocardial infarction than in subsequent periods (this is discussed further below).

3.1.2. **Building time-dependency into Markov transition probabilities**

The HIV case study used to illustrate Markov models in Chapter 2 assumed that all transition probabilities were fixed with respect to time. For example, the annual probability of dying when in the 'AIDS state' was the same regardless of how long the patient had been in that state. As for all modelling assumptions, this is a simplification of reality. The critical issue is whether the simplification is markedly at odds with reality and may generate potentially misleading results in terms of the cost-effectiveness of the options

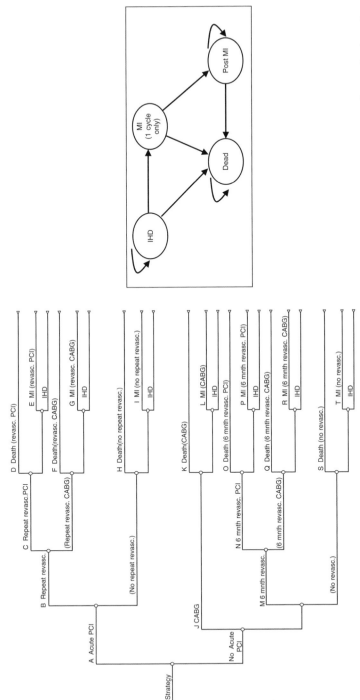

Fig. 3.1 Example of the use of a decision tree and Markov model within the same cost-effectiveness analysis, in the context of an evaluation of glycoprotein 2b/3a antagonists for acute coronary syndrome (Palmer et al. 2005). The left panel shows the decision tree and the right panel shows the Markov model used for extrapolation. Revasc: revascularization; PCI: percutaneous coronary intervention; IHD: ischaemic heart disease; MI: myocardial infarction; CABG: coronary artery bypass grafting; mnth: month

being compared. For those models where the assumption of constant transition probabilities is considered too strong, there are ways of letting some transition probabilities vary with time.

Types of time-dependency

To understand how this is possible, it is important to distinguish between two types of time-dependency in transition probabilities in Markov models; these are described below.

Probabilities that vary according to time in model. The simplest form of time-dependency in Markov models is where transition probabilities vary according to how long the cohort has been modelled. In other words, the probability of one or more transitions changes as the cohort ages. Returning to the HIV case study in Chapter 2, transitions to State D (i.e. the probability of dying) were assumed fixed with respect to time (Fig. 2.3, Table 2.2). However, it may be considered more appropriate to assume that, as the cohort ages, the annual probability of death increases. This would probably make more sense if the probability of death was divided into two: HIV/AIDS-specific mortality and other-case mortality. With such a division, it might be reasonable to have constant transition probabilities for the first, but to increase transition probabilities as the cohort ages for the second.

The starting age of the cohort should be explicitly stated, as this would typically be an important element in characterizing the individuals to whom the intervention applies, especially when its impact on mortality is being modelled. Furthermore, for cost-effectiveness modelling, the cohort should be homogeneous, as the decision problem is to establish the most cost-effective option for specifically defined groups of individuals. If the starting age of the cohort is known, then so is the age of the cohort at any cycle of the model, whatever the state. In order to implement age-dependent probabilities, therefore, it is simply necessary to have a unique transition probability for each cycle. This is shown in Table 3.1, which revises the transition probability matrix for the HIV case study shown in Table 2.2. Instead of one 'dead' state, there are now two: HIV/AIDS-related (State D) and other-cause (State E). Transitions to State E are assumed to be age-dependent as defined in the table below the main transition probability matrix. These age-dependent probabilities might be taken from national life tables. As the cycle number increases, so does the probability of moving to State E. As the transition probabilities need to sum to 1 horizontally, the probability of remaining in a given state for the next cycle has to allow for the age-dependent probability.

Probabilities which vary according to time in state. The second type of time-dependency relates to situations where a transition probability changes as

Table 3.1 Revised transition probability matrix for the HIV case study where transitions to a dead state vary with the age of the cohort. See Table 2.2 for initial transitions

	State A	State B	State C	State D	State E
State A	1 − 0.202 − 0.067 − 0.010 − P(age)	0.202	0.067	0.010	P(age)
State B	0.000	1 − 0.407 − 0.012 − P(age)	0.407	0.012	P(age)
State C	0.000	0.000	1 − 0.250 − P(age)	0.250	P(age)
State D	0.000	0.000	0.000	1.0	0.000
State E	0.000	0.000	0.000	0.000	1.0

P(age1)	P(age2)	P(age3)	P(age4)	P(age5)	P(age6)	P(age7)	P(age8)	P(age9)	P(age10)
0.001	0.001	0.002	0.003	0.003	0.005	0.005	0.006	0.006	0.007

States A, B and C are as defined in Fig. 2.3. State D is HIV/AIDS-specific mortality and State E is other-case mortality. The numbers in the table below the main transition probability matrix are the age-dependent probabilities of other-cause mortality over a 10-year period.

time in a state increases. As a result of the Markov assumption, this form of time-dependency is less straightforward to implement. In the HIV case study, it may be the case that the probability of dying while in the AIDS state increases as the time the patient has had AIDS increases. Ideally, it would be possible to increase the transition probability from State C to State D in Fig. 2.3 to reflect this. However, the Markov assumption is such that, once a patient has entered State C, the model cannot establish at which point they entered so it cannot 'keep track' of how long they have been in the state. Therefore, as currently structured, it would not be possible to implement this form of time-dependency between States C and D.

However, if it was the case that the probability of moving between State A and one or more of the other states in the model was considered to vary depending on how long the patient had been in State A, this could be implemented quite easily. This is because all patients start the model in State A at a given time point and, once they have left that state, they are unable to return. It is, therefore, always possible to keep track of how long any patient has been in State A. In this case, of course, making a transition probability dependent on time in state is exactly the same as making it dependent on the age of the cohort because they are in that state from the start of the model.

Using survival analysis to implement time-dependency

The example of time-dependency illustrated in Table 3.1 simply uses a 'look-up' table to define the time-dependent probabilities. This would be appropriate when data are readily presented in such a format in the literature or in routine statistics (e.g. routine life tables). It is often the case, however, that the relationship between a transition probability and time can be explicitly estimated from patient-level data. Such data would typically come from some sort of longitudinal study (e.g. a trial or cohort study) which has recorded the time to one or more events for each patient. The appropriate way of analysing such 'time to event' data is survival analysis.

The use of survival models in the medical field is widespread and well understood. Their key feature is that they can handle (noninformative) censoring that frequently occurs in follow-up studies – that is, observation ceases before some patients have experienced the event of interest. The most popular form of survival model is the semiparametric Cox proportional hazards model (Cox and Oakes 1984). As this form of model does not specify how the risk of an event changes over time (i.e. the functional form of the hazard function), its use to inform time-dependency in Markov models is limited.

Alternatively, parametric survivor functions can be employed and can be fitted in many popular statistical packages (Collett 1994). It is important to emphasize, however, that standard survival analyses are based on hazard rates, but Markov models employ transition probabilities. As summarized in Box 3.1, there are important differences between rates and probabilities that have to be recognized in decision analysis, although they can readily be translated one to the other (Miller and Homan 1994). An example of the importance of this distinction is when flexibility is required in terms of the cycle length in a Markov model. Moving, say, from a 1-year to a 6-month cycle length involves more than merely dividing the transition probabilities by 2. Rather, instantaneous rates need to be derived and, from that, 6-month probabilities calculated. Understanding the differences between rates and probabilities is particularly important in the context of survival analysis.

Fundamental relationships in survival analysis. In order to understand how to use survival analysis to derive transition probabilities, some important concepts in survival analysis need to be introduced. The first of these is a probability density function (pdf) for survival data, $f(t)$, with an associated cumulative density function:

$$F(t) = P(T \leq t)$$

Box 3.1 A summary of the distinction between rates and probabilities

Rates

The instantaneous potential for the occurrence of an event, expressed per number of patients at risk.

Rates can be added and subtracted.

Probabilities

A number ranging between 0 and 1.

Represents the likelihood of an event happening over a specific period of time.

It is possible to convert an instantaneous rate to a probability over a particular time period, if the rate is assumed to be constant over that period:

$$p = 1 - \exp\{-rt\}$$

where p is the probability, r is the rate and t is the time period of interest.

Similarly, it is possible to convert a probability over a period of time to a (constant) instantaneous rate:

$$r = - [\ln(1-P)]/t$$

For example, assume 100 patients are followed up for 5 years after which 20 have had a particular event. Hence the 5-year probability of the event is 0.2. Assuming a fixed rate with respect to time, what is the instantaneous event rate?

$$\text{Rate} = - [\ln(1-0.2)]/5 = 0.04463$$

It is then possible to calculate a 1-year probability of the event:

$$\text{1-year probability} = 1 - \exp(-0.04463 \times 1) = 0.043648$$

Note that this 1-year event probability is not the same as the 5-year event probability divided by 5.

which gives the cumulative probability of failure up to time t. The complement of this function is the survivor function, that is, the probability of surviving for a period of time greater than t:

$$S(t) = P(T > t) = 1 - F(t).$$

Note that it is, therefore, straightforward to relate $f(t)$ and $S(t)$

$$f(t) = \frac{dF(t)}{dt} = \frac{d(1 - S(t))}{dt} = -S'(t). \tag{3.1}$$

It is now possible to define the hazard function (where the hazard is a rate), which is the instantaneous chance of failure at time t, conditional on having survived to time t, or, algebraically:

$$h(t) = \lim_{\delta t \to 0} \frac{P(t + \delta t \geq T > t \mid T > t)}{\delta t}.$$

The standard rule for conditional probabilities is $P(A|B) = P(A \text{ and } B)/P(B)$ (see Chapter 2), so this can be re-written as:

$$h(t) = \lim_{\delta t \to 0} \frac{P(t + \delta t \geq T > t)}{\delta t} \cdot \frac{1}{S(t)}$$

$$= \frac{f(t)}{S(t)}. \tag{3.2}$$

We now define the cumulative hazard function:

$$H(t) = \int_0^t \frac{f(u)}{S(u)} du$$

noting that the cumulative hazard up to time t is not the same as the probability of failure up to time t which is given by $F(t)$. Using the result from eqn 3.1 and the standard rules of calculus, we can express the cumulative hazard as a function of the survivor function:

$$H(t) = -\int_0^t \frac{S'(t)}{S(t)}$$

$$= -\ln\{S(t)\}$$

or, alternatively, as the survivor function in terms of the cumulative hazard:

$$S(t) = \exp\{-H(t)\}. \tag{3.3}$$

Estimating discrete time transition probabilities from instantaneous hazard rates.
The relationship in eqn 3.3 is central to the process used to derive transition
probabilities for Markov models. Consider a very simple Markov model with
just two states: alive and dead. Therefore, only one transition probability needs
to be estimated: the transition to death. Define the length of the Markov cycle
as u and let the instantaneous hazard of death at time t be represented by $h(t)$,
as above. The challenge, therefore, is to estimate the appropriate discrete
transition probability between time-points $t - u$ and t, call this $tp(t_u)$ where t_u
indicates that t is now measured as integer multiples of the cycle length of the
model, u.

The baseline transition probability of the event of interest can simply be
defined as one minus the ratio of the survivor function at the end of the interval
to the survivor function at the beginning of the interval:

$$tp(t_u) = 1 - S(t)/S(t-u)$$

which can be rewritten in terms of the cumulative hazard (from eqn 3.3) as:

$$tp(t_u) = 1 - \exp\{-H(t)\}/\exp\{-H(t-u)\}$$
$$= 1 - \exp\{H(t-u) - H(t)\}. \tag{3.4}$$

To see why it is important to move from the arguably more simple specification of the transition probability as the ratio of two points on the survival
curve to the specification in eqn 3.4, consider the application of a treatment
effect. It is common to include treatment effects as multiplicative, perhaps as
relative risks, or in terms of treatment effects estimated directly from a
survival analysis, in terms of a hazard ratio. Such a treatment effect should not
be applied directly to the baseline transition *probability*; rather, the treatment
effect (call this τ) should instead be applied to the hazard *rate*. Therefore, if
eqn 3.4 represents the baseline transition probability in the absence of treatment, the treatment transition would be given by:

$$tp_\tau(t_u) = 1 - \exp\{\tau[H(t-u) - H(t)]\}$$
$$= 1 - \exp\{H(t-u) - H(t)\}^\tau$$
$$\neq 1 - \tau \cdot \exp\{H(t-u) - H(t)\}.$$

The last line above indicates that it would be incorrect to multiply the treatment effect by the baseline probability. To illustrate how these methods are
used with actual data to populate specific decision models, two examples are
described below.

Example 1: acute myocardial infarction in patients with NSTACS. As part of the process of populating the Markov model shown in Fig. 3.1 in the GPA example above (Palmer *et al.* 2005), patient-level time-to-event (survival) data were available from an observational study where the event was acute myocardial infarction. These data were from 916 patients with (non-ST elevation acute coronary syndrome NSTACS). The maximum follow-up time was 5 years and 51 events were reported during that time. The aim was to estimate the risk of acute myocardial infarction in a model with yearly transition probabilities and to extrapolate to a 10-year timeframe.

A parametric Weibull model was employed to model these data (Collett 1994; Carroll 2003). The Weibull pdf is given by:

$$f(t) = \lambda \gamma t^{\gamma-1} \exp\{-\lambda t^{\gamma}\}$$

where the λ parameter gives the scale of the distribution and the (ancillary) γ parameter defines the shape. From the fundamental relationships of survival analysis described above, we can easily divide the pdf into component parts:

$$h(t) = \lambda \gamma t^{\gamma-1}$$
$$S(t) = \exp\{-\lambda t^{\gamma}\}$$
$$H(t) = \lambda t^{\gamma}.$$

Fig. 3.2 shows different time-dependent hazard functions that can be modelled using the Weibull function. The shape of these alternative functions depends on the value of the γ parameter. For example, when γ is between

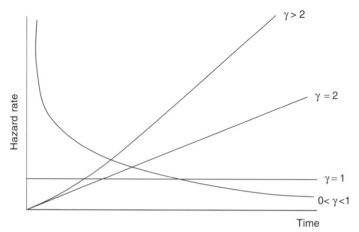

Fig. 3.2 Illustration of the different time-dependent hazard rates that can be generated with the Weibull model depending on the value of γ, the shape parameter (Collett 1994).

Table 3.2 STATA output for a Weibull regression to derive time-dependent
probabilities of acute myocardial infarction in patients with non-ST-elevation
acute coronary syndrome

Weibull regression – log relative-hazard form

No. subjects	916			No. obs		916
No. failures	52					
Time at risk*	1058651			LR chi² (0)		−0.00
Log likelihood	−262.00507			Prob > chi²		

	Coef.	SE	z	P > |z|	(95% Confidence interval)	
_cons	−8.028897	0.6855026	−11.71	0.000	−9.372457	−6.685336
/ln_p	−0.3040257	0.1268008	−2.40	0.016	−0.5525507	−0.0555008
p	0.7378419	0.0935589			0.5754801	0.9460113
1/p	1.355304	0.1718536			1.05707	1.73768

* Note that the unit of time for this regression model is measured in days.

0 and 1, the hazard rate falls over time. Also, the Weibull model nests the
exponential as a special case when $\gamma = 1$.

Table 3.2 shows the results of a Weibull survival analysis using the acute
myocardial infarction data based on the software package STATA v7.0.
It should be noted that, in the STATA output, the constant _cons is the $\ln(\lambda)$
value and $p = \gamma$. Note that the 'p' parameter in the table (equivalent to the
shape parameter γ in the exposition above) is less than 1 (and statistically
significantly so), indicating evidence for a decreasing hazard over time. Hence,
in the Markov model, it is possible to have transition probabilities to
the myocardial infarction state which decrease as cycles elapse. These yearly
transitions estimated from these data are given in Table 3.3. These are generated from the following equation, which is derived from the general form in
eqn 3.4 above, substituting the expression for the cumulative hazard from the
Weibull as given above:

$$tp(t_u) = 1 - \exp\left\{\lambda(t-u)^\gamma - \lambda t^\gamma\right\}.$$

Example 2: Cause-specific death from early breast cancer following surgery.
A patient-level data set was obtained from the Medical Oncology Unit at the
Churchill Hospital, Oxford, containing personal and clinical details of breast
cancer patients treated at this centre from 1986 onwards. Patients were
selected who had operable breast cancer, and who had at least 5 years of
follow-up information subsequent to initial surgery (maximum follow-up was
15 years). The aim was to predict death from early breast cancer for women
with different prognostic characteristics (Campbell *et al.* 2003).

Table 3.3 Estimated yearly transition probabilities to myocardial infarction, based on the Weibull model, in patients with non-ST-elevation acute coronary syndrome

Year	Transition probabilities (%)
1	2.47
2	1.68
3	1.46
4	1.34
5	1.25
6	1.19
7	1.14
8	1.1
9	1.06
10	1.03

An initial exploration of the model used the Weibull function, but found that the hypothesis of a constant hazard could not be rejected. Therefore, a straightforward exponential model (constant transition probabilities) was employed. The pdf for an exponential distribution is given by:

$$f(t) = \lambda \exp\{-\lambda t\}$$

and this can be split into component parts:

$$h(t) = \lambda$$
$$S(t) = \exp\{-\lambda t\}$$
$$H(t) = \lambda t.$$

The Oxford data were employed to estimate the baseline transition probabilities of breast cancer death in the absence of adjuvant therapy. Thus the baseline transitions were estimated as:

$$tp_0(t_u) = 1 - \exp\{\lambda(t-u) - \lambda t\}$$
$$= 1 - \exp\{-\lambda u\}$$

where $\ln(\lambda)$ is the linear predictor of covariates. This is consistent with the process of moving between the instantaneous (constant) rate and the transition probability, as described above and in Box 3.1. The exponential model represents the standard assumption in Markov models: the hazard rate and transition probability are fixed with respect to time.

3.1.3. **Relaxing the Markov assumption**

Chapter 2 introduced the concept of the Markov assumption, which relates to the fact that, in determining future transitions in such a model, there is no memory of what has happened to 'patients' in the past. In many situations, this feature of Markov models will not be a limiting factor. However, this may not be the case in modelling some diseases and technologies. Given the computational ease of using cohort models, it would be desirable to be able to relax the Markov assumption while retaining the cohort feature. Figure 2.5 illustrated the Markov assumption using the example of a model evaluating cancer therapy. The key feature of this model was that once a patient has been treated for either local or regional recurrence of their cancer and entered the 'remission' state, the model is unable to take into account the details of those past events in determining future transitions.

One way to 'build memory' into the model is to add additional states. This is illustrated in Fig. 3.3 using the example introduced in Fig. 2.5. Compared with the model structure shown in Fig. 2.5, which had one state representing remission following treatment for a cancer recurrence, the revised model now has six. The use of multiple 'remission' states allows the model to reflect that future transitions (here, the risk of death), costs and health-related quality of life may differ according to two factors: when a patient was treated for a cancer recurrence (in terms of time since initial treatment or start of the model); and whether their recurrence was local or regional to the initial primary tumour.

The first of these is a form of time-dependency with the future transitions, costs and health-related quality of life dependent on how long a patient has been in remission. As discussed in Section 3.1.2, this form of time-dependency

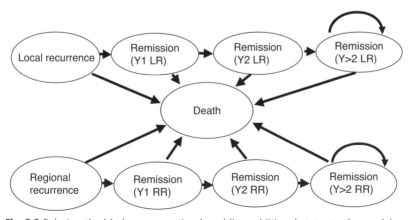

Fig. 3.3 Relaxing the Markov assumption by adding additional states to the model shown in Fig. 2.5.

cannot be implemented in the standard Markov model in Fig. 2.5 because it depends on time in a state that is not the initial state in the model. The addition of extra states to the model makes this form of time-dependency possible because 'memory' is added. The time-dependency is characterized in terms of two tunnel states where patients remain for only one cycle (here, 1 year), during which they may have different transition probabilities, costs and health-related quality of life to the other. If they survive the tunnel states, patients go into a third remission state, at which point future transitions, costs and health-related quality of life may be different from those in the tunnel states and are constant with respect to time.

Hence the tunnel state is a way of implementing time-dependency by adding memory to a Markov model. Such models have been referred to as semi-Markov processes (Billingham *et al.* 1999). If extensive time-dependency is required, however, a large number of tunnel states may be necessary. In such situations, programming the model in a spreadsheet can be very difficult. One way around this is to use a mathematical programming language such as R, which facilitates multidimensional transition probability matrices (Ihaka and Gentleman 1996). This sort of approach has been used in applied cost-effectiveness studies, although it is uncommon. For example, in a recent cost-effectiveness analysis of new treatments for epilepsy in adults, a semi-Markov model was used, reflecting the fact that available evidence indicated the probability of treatment failure reduced with time (Hawkins *et al.* 2005*a*; Hawkins *et al.* 2005*b*). To implement this using standard tunnel states would have been too complicated to program in a spreadsheet, not least because the model related to sequences of treatments rather than individual therapies. Therefore, the model was implemented in R using a transition probability matrix with three dimensions: one for the state where the patient starts the cycle, one for the state where they finish the cycle and one for number of cycles in the starting state. Multidimensional matrices can be used to reflect other types of 'patient history' into cohort models such as previous events.

3.2. **Patient-level simulation models**

3.2.1. **The features of patient-level simulation**

Although cohort models predominate in cost-effectiveness modelling, some studies focus on modelling the progression of individual patients through the model rather than a cohort. These patient-level simulation models (sometimes termed microsimulations or individual sampling models) can be attractive when the assumptions of cohort models (in particular, Markov chains) prove too limiting. As individuals are moved through the model one at a time, rather than as proportions of a cohort, the memoryless feature of the Markov does not apply. Specifically, with patient-level simulation, the accumulating history of the patient can be used to determine transitions, costs and health-related quality of life.

This can be seen in the context of the cancer model illustrated in Fig. 2.5. A given individual patient can experience, say, a local recurrence 3 years after initial surgery. They can then go into the remission state, during which time they are at risk of further recurrence and death. If the understanding of the disease suggests that once in the remission state, a patient's risks of further recurrence and death are a function of whether they had a local or regional recurrence, and the time since that recurrence, additional states need to be added to the standard Markov model.

For patient-level simulation, the fact that patients are tracked individually means that it is possible for the model to reflect a patient's history (in terms, for example, of details of and times since past events). There are several alternative forms of this sort of model (Davies 1985; Barton *et al.* 2004). For example, some models are similar to the standard Markov model in using states, discrete time periods and transition probabilities. Discrete-event simulation, however, is structured around how long the individual patient remains in a state rather than the probability of moving to another state. More detailed overviews of the use of patient-level simulation models in economic evaluation are available (Karnon 2003; Barton *et al.* 2004).

There are, however, disadvantages to the use of patient-level simulation. The first is that they can be more demanding of data. That is, if various aspects of patient history are used to determine future prognosis, then the model will require input parameters, which are conditional on those patient characteristics. For example, for the cancer model discussed above, it would be necessary to estimate the risk of death as a function of time in remission and dependent on the type of recurrence the patient had experienced. There is another perspective on this apparent drawback. Sometimes a large and detailed dataset is available in a given area, and patient-level simulation can be used to reflect the richness of the data. Models developed in such a way can then be used to address a range of specific decision problems in the disease area as they emerge. This is a different premise for the development of decision models than is usually the case when a decision analysis is undertaken to inform a specific decision problem at a particular point in time.

An example of a patient-level simulation used to model a specific dataset and hence to become a 'generic' model available for a range of decision problems is the UKPDS Outcomes Model (Clarke *et al.* 2004; http://www.dtu.ox.ac.uk/index.html?maindoc=/outcomesmodel/; accessed June 2006). A schematic of the model's structure is presented in Fig. 3.4. This is a patient-level simulation

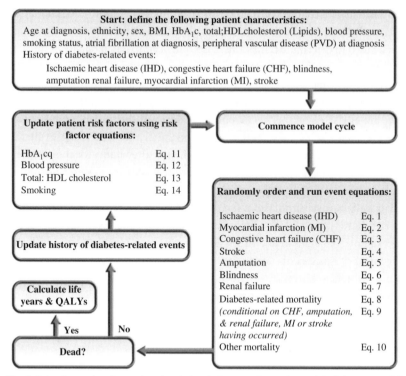

Fig. 3.4 A schematic of a patient-level simulation used as a 'generic' diabetes model using data from the UKPDS Outcomes Model (Clarke *et al.* 2004).

based on 3642 individual patients from the United Kingdom Prospective Diabetes Study (UKPDS Study Group 1998) which is implemented as a series of interrelated parametric equations. The value of patient-level simulation in this case is that it provides a flexible way of reflecting that patients are at competing risk of seven diabetes-related complications over time (e.g. renal failure, myocardial infarction, blindness and stroke), and that experiencing one of these events may change the patient's risk of experiencing one of the others in the future. When a model is parameterized using individual patient data from a single study, it is important that all relevant evidence has been used. As discussed in Chapter 1, this can be regarded as a requirement of decision making.

A second potential drawback with patient-level simulation is the computational burden. To estimate expected costs and expected effects in such models requires a large cohort of patients to be simulated. Compared with the cohort simulation, this can be time-consuming, but such models can allow a level of complexity to be captured in their structure that may not be possible with cohort models.

A third limitation, which is related to the second, is the flexibility of these models to assess uncertainty. Chapter 2 outlined the key concepts in uncertainty analysis in decision modelling (see Box 2.1), and these are further developed in Chapter 4. Patient-level simulations are primarily focused on modelling variability in events (and hence costs and outcomes) between patients. Their rationale is that, by more fully reflecting the complexity of between-patient variability, a more appropriate estimate of expected cost-effectiveness will result. There is less flexibility in these models, however, in assessing parameter uncertainty. A given set of simulations (e.g. 10 000 individual patients) will be based on a set of fixed input parameters. The conventional way in which the implications of uncertainty in those parameters is assessed in patient simulation models is simple sensitivity analysis – that is, to change a small number of parameter values and consider the change in results. For larger models, even this can represent a computational burden, as the full set of simulations would typically have to be run for all changes in the input parameters.

The major burden, however, comes when the joint uncertainty in all parameters (and its implications for decision uncertainty) is assessed using probabilistic sensitivity analysis (PSA) (Briggs *et al.* 2003; Claxton *et al.* 2005). These methods are described fully in Chapters 4 and 5. In the context of patient-level simulation, a full assessment of parameter and decision uncertainty using PSA will require two levels of simulation: one level based on fixed parameters to estimate a single expected value; and the second to sample from a distribution of possible input values. With, say, 10 000 simulations for the two levels of simulations, this would result in 100 million individual simulations. This is only likely to be feasible for a small proportion of patient-level simulation models implemented in a fast programming language. As discussed further in Chapter 4, even if the focus of a model is to estimate expected costs and effects, when a model exhibits a nonlinear relationship between inputs and outputs (as it true, for example, with a Markov model), simulating across the distributions of the parameters using probabilistic methods is necessary to get appropriate expectations.

A shortcut to avoid this time-consuming computation has been developed using a statistical model called a Gaussian process (Stevenson *et al.* 2004), although this is yet to be widely used. Methods are also being developed to use analysis of variance (ANOVA) methods to make PSA more practical in patient-level simulation methods (O'Hagan *et al.* 2005). The simulation associated with undertaking value of information analysis (see Chapters 6 and 7) represents an even greater magnitude of computational burden.

3.2.2. **Examples of a patient-level simulations and comparisons with cohort models**

Patient-level simulation models are quite widely used to evaluate changes in health service organization. For example, a discrete-event simulation was used to assess the cost-effectiveness of reorganizing surgical and anaesthesia services (Stahl *et al.* 2004). The model sought to balance changes in safety (in terms of avoidable medical errors) with gains in efficiency (in terms of throughput) as a result of increasing patient volume. The authors argued for the advantages of discrete-event simulation for their research in terms of the need to reflect the fact that the probability of events, the duration of processes and the rate at which patients enter the model are stochastic processes. In addition, this sort of model allows patients to interact or compete for finite resources which, in turn, can stimulate further effects in the model.

Patient-level simulation models are also being used for the economic evaluation of medical interventions. An example is a model looking at the cost-effectiveness of population screening for *Helicobacter pylori* infection to prevent gastric cancer and peptic ulcer disease (Roderick *et al.* 2003). A schematic of the model is shown in Fig. 3.5. Unlike the usual Markov-type model, the 'states' in the model reflect both health-related events (e.g. gastric cancer) and health service delivery (e.g. give triple therapy). The authors use the model to simulate a series of cohorts of individual patients: a prevalence cohort and then a series of incidence cohorts. The authors do not describe why the use of patient-level simulation has major advantages over cohort modelling in their research. The potential limitations of the methods in handling uncertainty are clearly demonstrated, in that only one or two parameters were varied at a time. Furthermore, although the authors emphasize the major parameter uncertainties in the model, the use of formal value of information methods would be difficult to achieve, and certainly was not attempted in the model.

There is a small literature comparing cohort models and patient-level simulations. One study compared these two types of model in their predictions of 20-year events in patients with type 2 diabetes (Brown *et al.* 2000). The authors compared 12 starting cohorts (or patients) in terms of baseline characteristics such as age, blood sugar and blood pressure. Both models generated clinically realistic results. The comparison indicated that the cohort model predicted higher rates of mortality and myocardial infarction, but fewer strokes. The extent to which this comparison was able show which type of model is superior was, however, limited by the fact that, in addition to different model structures, they also used different evidence and assumptions.

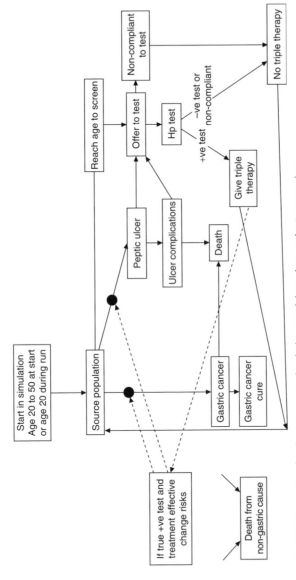

Fig. 3.5 Schematic of a discrete event simulation model used to evaluate screening for *Helicobacter pylori* (Roderick *et al.* 2003).

In another study, a Markov model and discrete-event simulation were compared in the context of a cost-effectiveness analysis of chemotherapy plus tamoxifen versus tamoxifen alone in node-positive breast cancer in post-menopausal women under the age of 65 years (Karnon 2003). Unlike the comparison of models in type 2 diabetes, the evidence used in the two models was the same. As a result of the differing characteristics of the Markov and discrete-event models, however, some of the assumptions differed. For example, the Markov model had a cycle length of one month, but the discrete-event simulation had a minimum time in a state of one month; in addition, survival times with metastatic breast cancer assumed a constant mortality rate but the discrete-event simulation used time-specific rates available in the literature. Many of the structural assumptions in the two models were, however, the same. Probabilistic sensitivity analysis was undertaken on both types of model, but the differences in computational burden were clear as the simulations for the Markov model took 1 hour and the discrete-event simulation took 3 days. The results of the two types of model were remarkably similar in terms of both the direction of the differences and the absolute values. The incremental cost per quality-adjusted life-year (QALY) gained for the Markov model was £3365 compared with £3483 with the discrete-event simulation. In terms of uncertainty, the cost-effectiveness acceptability curves (see Chapter 5) generated by the two model types were very similar. Despite the similarity in overall results, however, the author emphasized that there were important differences in the models but that, in terms of the final results, these tended to cancel each other out. A key difference was in the estimated survival times once a patient had developed metastatic cancer.

In selecting between a cohort model and a patient-level simulation, it is important to be aware of their strengths and weaknesses. The methods literature comparing the two types of model is small, and further research of this type is required. A key consideration in the selection is that all models are approximations of reality, so how far should a model be pushed in reflecting the features of a disease or the interventions? Patient-level simulations may go further in this respect, but this comes at a cost in terms of data requirements and computational burden. When alternative types of model have been developed for a given decision problem, it is quite straightforward to see whether the patient-level models are worth their extra 'cost' in terms of whether the results and conclusions differ. In the case of the Karnon comparison described above, the simpler Markov model would have sufficed, as the results were very similar between the two model types (Karnon 2003). However, assessing potential differences in results from different model types before the models are constructed is more difficult. From a pragmatic viewpoint, the analyst needs to get a clear idea of the sort of structural features that the model should exhibit, and assess how far a standard cohort-type model will take them in reflecting that structure. If such a model falls short of the requirements, there needs to be a consideration of whether building on the cohort concept will bridge the gap, for example, using additional states, time-dependent probabilities or a semi-Markov process. If the enhanced cohort model still falls short of what is required for an 'adequate structure', then patient-level simulation may be necessary if the computational burden involved with reflecting parameter and decision uncertainty can be dealt with.

3.3. **Static versus dynamic models in infectious disease**

An important area where different types of model can potentially have a major impact on results is in the economic evaluation of interventions for infectious diseases, in particular evaluations of vaccination programmes. However, the key distinction in this area is not between cohort models and patient-level simulations, but between dynamic and static models (Edmunds *et al.* 1999; Brisson and Edmunds 2003). Most models used in the economic evaluation of vaccination programmes are static, in that they assume that the rate of infection among a susceptible population is fixed. Dynamic models more accurately reflect the reality of infectious diseases, in that the rate of infection is a function of the number of infected individuals in the community. Therefore, dynamic models explicitly allow for the effects of herd immunity in a way that cannot be achieved with a static model. Furthermore, as described in Chapter 2, static models will typically focus on a cohort that ages as it progresses through the model. Dynamic models, on the other hand, are run over many years on the basis of multiple cohorts.

Brisson and Edmunds used the example of an economic evaluation of a simplified infant varicella vaccination programme to highlight the major differences in results that can be generated by these two types of model (Brisson and Edmunds 2003). The number of infected cases was predicted over time with the two types of model (see Fig. 3.6). Fully reflecting the dynamic nature of the disease with respect to herd immunity results in three distinct phases. These are marked as 2, 3 and 4 in Fig. 3.6a, with period 1 being the prevaccination period. The first phase is referred to as the 'honeymoon period' shortly after the vaccination programme begins, when the number of susceptibles falls sufficiently to prevent endemic transmission and the number of infected cases is very low. The second is the post-honeymoon epidemic,

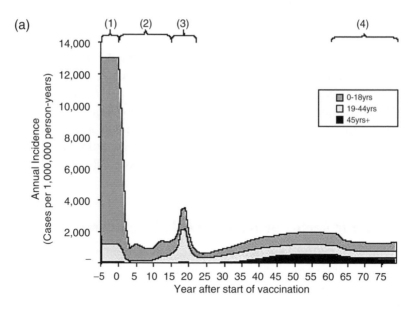

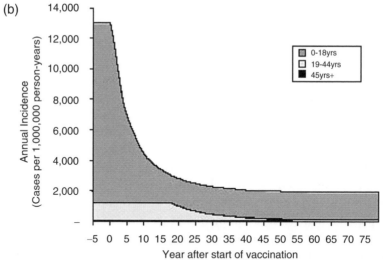

Fig. 3.6 Comparison of the number cases of varicella infection over time, following the introduction of an infant vaccination programme. (a) Shows the predicted results with a dynamic model which is able explicitly to reflect herd immunity; and (b) shows the predictions with a standard static model (Brisson and Edmunds 2003).

when the number of susceptibles increases (through births) above a threshold that results in an increase in infections to epidemic level. The third period is the postvaccination endemic equilibrium where a long-term equilibrium is reached with lower infection levels than prior to the vaccination programme. The static model cannot capture these three distinct periods (Fig. 3.5b) and, as a result, underestimates the number of infections avoided (in the example in the paper, by 10 million over 80 years for England and Wales). The difference between the two models is due to the static model's inability to reflect herd immunity, the effect of which depends on the extent of continuing infection in the community. Therefore, for decision problems relating to infectious diseases where herd immunity is important, dynamic models are essential. It is possible to develop both cohort and patient-level simulation versions of dynamic models.

3.4. **Summary**

For a given decision problem, there is a need for the analyst to decide how to reflect the essential features of a disease, and the impact of interventions. This has to be done in a way that recognizes that all models are approximations of reality. It is not possible to approach this structuring process in a formulaic way. Rather, judgements need to be taken in such a way as to find an appropriate balance between two key attributes. The first is to provide clinical 'face validity' in the sense that assumptions used in the model are plausible given what is known about the disease and the interventions. The second is that model needs to be fit for purpose in terms of its outputs. That is, it needs to provide estimates of expected costs and effects of all relevant options over an appropriate time horizon. It also needs to be sufficiently tractable to facilitate detailed sensitivity analysis including probabilistic methods.

3.5. **Exercise: constructing a Markov model of total hip replacement**

3.5.1. **Overview**

The purpose of this exercise is to build another Markov model in Excel. The model will illustrate a number of facets of model building in the Markov framework that complement the HIV/AIDS model example from Chapter 2. Of particular interest is the use of time-dependent transition functions to represent probabilities. The exercise will get you to construct two types of transition probabilities: time-varying transitions from a life table, and time-varying transitions estimated from a parametric survival model.

The step-by-step guide below will take you through a number of stages of developing the model, which is based on a simplified version of a published cost-effectiveness model (Briggs *et al.* 2004). These steps are:

1. Preparing parameters and naming cells.
2. Parametric time-dependent transitions from a survival analysis.
3. Life table transitions for background mortality.
4. Building a Markov model for the standard prosthesis.
5. Adapting the model for a new prosthesis.
6. Estimating cost-effectiveness (deterministically).

Before beginning the exercise take a moment to familiarize yourself with the Excel template for the exercise, '*Exercise 3.5 – template.xls*'. The first worksheet in the workbook <*Model Figure*> contains the overall structure of the model you are about to build. It will be worth spending a little time familiarizing yourself with this figure; it is also presented in Fig. 3.7. The figure contains a state transition diagram of the four-state Markov model you will be building and contains a key to the different parameters of the model, which are colour-coded into three categories: transition probabilities, state costs and state utilities. The model itself is constructed across a number of sheets. There are separate sheets for the parameters of the model and the final analysis, for the survival analysis used to estimate prosthesis failure rates, for each of the Markov model

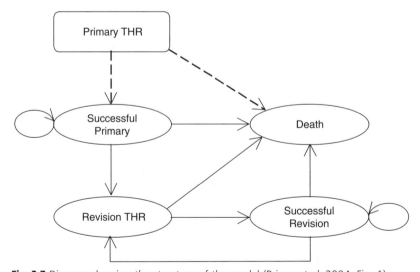

Fig. 3.7 Diagram showing the structure of the model (Briggs *et al.* 2004, Fig. 1).

arms of the model and for the life tables used for mortality rates. Of course, there are many ways to structure models – much being down to personal preference. However, we hope that you will find that our chosen way of presenting the model does not deviate too much from your own preferences!

3.5.2. **Step-by-step guide**

All cells for you to complete in the exercise are coloured yellow. However, make sure that you also pay attention to the content of the surrounding cells, as although these may not require changes, they provide important information, much of which you will have to use.

1. Preparing parameters and naming cells

The aim of this section of the exercise is to prepare the *<Parameters>* worksheet to facilitate the use of parameter names throughout the rest of the modelling exercise. On opening the worksheet you will see that much of the work has been done for you, including entry of patient characteristics (linked to the *<Analysis>* worksheet), the inclusion of standard discounting rates, and the cost of the two prostheses that we are seeking to evaluate. This section will guide you through the completion of the parameter information for the (constant) transition probabilities, the state costs, the state utilities and the naming of parameters.

 i. We will start with the three transition probabilities that will be assumed to be constant in the model: the operative mortality rates and the re-revision rate parameters in cells B16:B18. We will assume that the operative mortality is 2 per cent for both primary and revision procedures and that the re-revision rate is 4 per cent per annum. Enter these values now.

Note that we will be returning to the time-dependent risk of prosthesis failure (revision risk) below, so for the moment leave B22:B27 blank.

 ii. Now we deal with the costs in the model. Note that the costs of the prostheses (standard and new) have already been entered for you. That leaves the costs for the states of the model. However, the state cost for the primary procedure is assumed to be the same irrespective of the implant – we therefore leave this out (as it is received by both arms and nets out of the analysis). For the purpose of this model we also assume that there is no ongoing cost to the health service if people have a successful implant in place. Therefore the only cost to consider at this point is the cost of the revision procedure itself. This has been estimated as £5294 and this should be entered into cell B33.

   iii. The quality-of-life utilities of a year spent in each of the model health states has been estimated to be 0.85, 0.75 and 0.30 for the successful primary, successful revision and revision states respectively. Enter these values into cells B41:B43.

Notice that the *<Parameters>* worksheet has been structured with columns for 'name', 'value', and 'description' for each parameter. We will exploit the fact that we can automate the naming of parameters by giving cells the name of the label in an adjacent cell. Naming is very powerful – it is much easier to remember parameter names than cell references and this means that mistakes are less likely to happen.

   iv. Highlight the 'name' and 'value' of the patient characteristics (i.e. highlight cells A8:B9). Now choose *Insert > Name > Create* from the menu bar. Excel will recognize that you may be trying to create names from adjacent labels in the left column, so answer 'OK' to the pop-up box.

   v. Check that the naming has been successful by selecting, in turn, cells B8 and B9. If you have successfully named these cells, then, when a cell is selected, you will see the name appear in the 'name box' at the top left of the screen immediately above the workbook.

   vi. Now continue to name all of the parameter cells on this worksheet down to row 43. (Note that you can even name the cells of the revision rate regression parameters that we have not yet entered.)

An alternative way of naming cells is to use *Insert > Name > Define* from the menu bar, which allows individual cell/area naming. We will use this method in the next section for naming a column, however it is much quicker to input a large number of parameter names using the automatic method.

2. Parametric time-dependent transitions from a survival analysis

If you open the *<Hazard function>* worksheet you will see the output of a regression analysis on prosthesis failure. A parametric Weibull model was fitted to patient level survival time data to estimate this function. The regression model shows that prosthesis survival time is significantly related to age, sex and type of prosthesis (new versus standard). In addition, the significance of the gamma parameter indicates that there is an important time-dependency to the risk of failure, which increases over time.

Note that the estimation of this regression model was undertaken on the log hazard scale. We therefore have to exponentiate the results to get the actual hazard rate. The exponents of the individual coefficients are interpreted as hazard ratios (column E). For example, the new prosthesis has a hazard ratio of 0.26, indicating that it is a much lower hazard compared with the standard prosthesis.

Take a moment to understand this survival model. If you are having trouble with the appropriate interpretation then do re-read the appropriate section on pages 50-56 – we are about to implement this model and you may struggle if you are not clear on the interpretation from the start.

i. To start with, generate a link from the *<Parameters>* worksheet (cells B22:B24 and B26:B27) to the corresponding results of the survival analysis on the *<Hazard function>* worksheet (cells C6:C10). Remember that these values are on the log hazard scale.

ii. We now want to calculate the lambda value of Weibull distribution (this, together with the gamma parameter, enables us to specify the baseline hazard). In estimating a standard survival analysis, it is the log of the lambda parameter that is a linear sum of the coefficients multiplied by the explanatory variables. Therefore, to get the value of log lambda, multiply the coefficients of age and sex (cells B23:B24) by the age and sex characteristics (cells B8:B9) and add together, not forgetting to also add the constant term (cell B22). Enter this formula into cell B25.

iii. Remember that the parameters in cells B25:B27 are on the log scale. Exponentiate each of these cells to give the value of the lambda and gamma parameters of the Weibull distribution and the hazard ratio for the new prosthesis compared with the standard.

Note that what we have estimated so far are the constant parts of the parametric Weibull hazard function. The task now is to make this time-dependent – we cannot do this on the *<Parameters>* worksheet – instead this must be done on the model worksheet itself. Open the *<Standard>* worksheet that contains the outline of the Markov model for the standard prosthesis.

In preparation for building the Markov model we are going to specify the time-dependent transition probability for prosthesis failure. Note the (annual) cycle is listed in column A for 60 years – this is our time variable. Recall from earlier that the cumulative hazard rate for the Weibull is given by:

$$H(t) = \lambda t^{\gamma}$$

and that the time-dependent transition probability (for a yearly cycle length and time measured in years) is given by:

$$tp(t) = 1 - \exp\{H(t-1) - H(t)\}$$
$$= 1 - \exp\{\lambda(t-1)^{\gamma} - \lambda t^{\gamma}\}$$
$$= 1 - \exp\{\lambda\left[(t-1)^{\gamma} - t^{\gamma}\right]\}.$$

iv. Use this formula to calculate the time-dependent transition probability for the standard prosthesis (referred to in the spreadsheet as 'revision risk') using the cycle number for the time variable and the lambda and gamma parameters already defined (you can now refer to these by name). Remember that Excel recognizes only one type of parenthesis, whereas the formula above uses different types for clarity.

v. Finally, in preparation for using these time-dependent transitions select this vector (cells C7:C66) and use the *Insert > Name > Define* pull-down menu to label the vector 'standardRR'.

You have just implemented a relatively sophisticated use of survival analysis to model a time-dependent transition in a Markov model. Note that it only works because we will be using this time-dependent transition from the initial state of the model, that is, we know exactly how long subjects have spent in the initial model state. Take a moment to make sure you understand what you have just implemented and the limitations on its use in a Markov framework.

3. Life table transitions for background mortality

We can still employ time-dependent transitions in other model states providing the time-dependency relates to time in the model rather than time in the state itself. This is the case for a background mortality rate, for example, which depends on the age of a subject rather than which state of the model they are in. In this section we will illustrate the use of a time-dependent transition to model background mortality in the model from a life table.

Open the *<Life tables>* worksheet and familiarize yourself with the contents. Rows 3–9 contain figures on age–sex specific mortality rates taken from a standard life table, published as deaths per thousand per year. These are converted to the corresponding annual probabilities in rows 14–20. Notice the addition of the 'Index' column – the reason for this will become apparent.

i. As a first step, name the table containing the transition probabilities 'Lifetable' taking care to include the index, but not the header row of labels (i.e. cells C15:E20).

You now need to familiarize yourself with the VLOOKUP(…) function in Excel – it would be a good idea to look up the function in Excel's help files. Also open the *<Standard>* worksheet and note that the time-dependent background mortality is to be entered in column E (labelled 'Death Risk').

ii. Use the VLOOKUP(…) command nested within in an IF(…) function in order to choose a value to be entered in the 'Death Risk' column based on the age and sex of the patient at that point in time.

Hints: you need to use two VLOOKUP(...) functions within the IF(...) statement dependent on the value of the sex of the subject (cell C9 on the <Parameters> worksheet). You have to add starting age to the cycle number to get current age which is used as the index in the VLOOKUP(...) function.

   iii. In preparation for using this newly entered information name the vector E7:E66 'mr' (for mortality rate).

You have now implemented all three key types of transition probability: constant, time-dependent (function) and time-dependent (tabular).

4. Building a Markov model for the standard prosthesis

Having specified the time-dependent transition parameters on the <Standard> worksheet we can now proceed to construct the Markov model proper. Initially, we are concerned only with generating the Markov trace, that is, showing the numbers of patients that are in any one state at any one time. This is the concern of columns G to L with H to K representing the four main model states, G represents the initial procedure, and K provides a check (as the sum across G to K must always equal the size of the original cohort).

The first step in building the Markov model is to define the transition matrix. This proceeds in exactly the same way as the HIV/AIDS example from Chapter 2.

   i. Start by defining the transition matrix in terms of the appropriate variable names, just as done for the HIV/AIDS model, using the information given in the state transition diagram of Fig. 3.7.

   ii. Use the transition matrix to populate the Markov model. This will involve representing the transitions between the different states represented in columns G to K. (You might want to review the hints given in Chapter 2 as to how to go about this). Remember not to use a remainder for the final (dead) state and then to check that all states sum to one in column L to make sure all people in your cohort are accounted for.

   iii. When you think you have the first row correct, copy this row down to the 59 rows below. If your check in column L is still looking good, then you have most likely done it correctly.

Now that we have the Markov trace, we can calculate the cost and effects for each cycle of the model.

   iv. In column M, calculate the cost of each cycle of the model (this is just the number of people in each state multiplied by the state cost).

Don't forget to include the cost discount rate and the cost of the original prosthesis in row 6.

v. In column N, calculate the life years. By doing this without quality adjustment or discounting, this column can be used to calculate life expectancy (which is often useful, although not in this example).

vi. In column O, calculate quality-adjusted life years by cycle. Again, don't forget to discount.

vii. Finally, in row 68, sum the columns and divide by 1000 to get the per patient predictions of cost, life expectancy and QALYs for this arm of the model. Use the automatic naming feature to generate the names given in row 67.

5. Adapting the model for a new prosthesis

Having constructed the standard prosthesis Markov model from scratch, it would be tedious to have to repeat much of the same to create the new prosthesis arm model. Instead we will adapt the standard model.

i. In the *<Standard>* worksheet, select the topmost left-hand corner cell (the one without a row or column label) – this highlights the whole worksheet. Copy the worksheet and highlight the same area on the <NP1> worksheet. Now paste and you should have an exact duplicate model ready to adapt.

ii. Firstly, we must introduce the treatment effect of the new prosthesis. This is easily achieved as the treatment effect reduces the baseline (standard) hazard ratio by the factor RRnp1 (a value of 26 per cent). Therefore apply this treatment effect parameter RRnp1 to the expression in column C taking care to reduce the hazard rate by this factor, not the probability (see page 53).

iii. Now rename the revision risk vector from 'standardRR' to 'np1RR'.

iv. Now update cells H7 and I7 to refer to np1RR rather than standard RR and copy this adjustment down to the 59 rows below.

v. Update cell M6 to refer to the cost of the new prosthesis rather than the standard prosthesis.

vi. Finally, update the labels in row 67 to an NP1 prefix and use the automatic naming feature to rename the row 68 cells below.

You should now have successfully adapted the Markov model to generate results for the cost, life expectancy and QALYs associated with using the new prosthesis.

6. Estimating cost-effectiveness (deterministically)

The final section of this exercise is very straightforward. We simply want to bring all the results together onto the <*Analysis*> worksheet for easy viewing.

    i. On the <*Analysis*> worksheet, link the cells for costs and QALYs for the two different models using the named results cells.

    ii. Calculate the incremental cost, incremental effect and the ICER.

That's it! Your Markov model is now complete. Have a play with the patient characteristics to see how these influence the results. Make sure you are clear in your own mind why patient characteristics influence the results. We will be returning to this issue of heterogeneity in Chapters 4 and 5.

References

Barton, P., Bryan, S. and Robinson, S. (2004) 'Modelling in the economic evaluation of health care: selecting the appropriate approach', *Journal of Health Services Research and Policy*, 9: 110–118.

Billingham, L. J., Abrams, K. R. and Jones, D. R. (1999) 'Methods for the analysis of quality-of-life and survival data in health technology assessment', *Health Technology Assessment*, 3 (entire issue).

Briggs, A. H., Ades, A. E. and Price, M. J. (2003) 'Probabilistic sensitivity analysis for decision trees with multiple branches: Use of the Dirichlet distribution in a Bayesian framework', *Medical Decision Making*, 23: 341–350.

Briggs A, Sculpher M, Dawson J, Fitzpatrick R, Murray D, Malchau H. (2004) 'Are new cemented prostheses cost-effective? A comparison of the Spectron and the Charnley', *Applied Health Economics* & *Health Policy*, 3: 78–89.

Brisson, M. and Edmunds, W. J. (2003) 'Economic evaluation of vaccination programs: the impact of herd-immunity', *Medical Decision Making*, 23: 76–82.

Brown, J. B., Palmer, A. J., Bisgaard, P., Chan, W., Pedula, K. and Russell, A. (2000) 'The Mt. Hood challenge: cross-testing two diabetes simulation models', *Diabetes Research and Clinical Practice*, 50 (Suppl. 3): S57–S64.

Campbell, H. E., Gray, A. M., Briggs, A. H. and Harris, A. (2003) 'Cost-effectiveness of using different prognostic information and decision criteria to select women with early breast cancer for adjuvant systemic therapy. Health Economists' Study Group Conference, Canterbury, July.

Carroll, K. J. (2003) 'On the use and utility of the Weibull model in the analysis of survival data', *Controlled Clinical Trials*, 24: 682–701.

Clarke, P. M., Gray, A. M., Briggs, A., Farmer, A. J., Fenn, P., Stevens, R. J., *et al.* (2004) 'A model to estimate the lifetime health outcomes of patients with type 2 diabetes: the United Kingdom Prospective Diabetes Study (UKPDS) Outcomes Model', *Diabetologia*, 47: 1747–1759.

Claxton, K., Sculpher, M., McCabe, C., Briggs, A., Akehurst, R., Buxton, M., *et al.* (2005) 'Probabilistic sensitivity analysis for NICE technology assessment: not an optional extra', *Health Economics*, 14: 339–347.

Collett, D. (1994) *Modelling survival data in medical research*. London, Chapman and Hall/CRC.

Cox, D. R. and Oakes, D. (1984) *Analysis of survival data*. London, Chapman & Hall.

Davies, R. (1985) 'An assessment of models of a health system', *Journal of the Operational Research Society*, 36: 679–687.

Edmunds, W. J., Medley, G. F. and Nokes, D. J. (1999) 'Evaluating the cost-effectiveness of vaccination programmes: a dynamic perspective', *Statistics in Medicine*, 18: 3263–3282.

Hawkins, N., Epstein, D., Drummond, M., Wilby, J., Kainth, A., Chadwick, D., *et al.* (2005a) 'Assessing the cost-effectiveness of new pharmaceuticals in epilepsy in adults: the results of a probabilistic decision model', *Medical Decision Making* 25: 493–510.

Hawkins, N., Sculpher, M. J. and Epstein, D. (2005b) 'Cost-effectiveness analysis of treatments for chronic disease – using R to incorporate time-dependency of treatment response', *Medical Decision Making* 25: 511–519.

Hollenberg, P. (1984) 'Markov cycle trees: a new representation for complex Markov processes'. Abstract from the Sixth Annual Meeting of the Society for Medical Decision Making, *Medical Decision Making*, 4.

Ihaka, R. and Gentleman, R. (1996) 'R: A language for data analysis and graphics', *Journal of Computational and Graphical Statistics*, 5: 299–314.

Karnon, J. (2003) 'Alternative decision modelling techniques for evaluation of health care technologies: Markov processes verses discrete event simulation', *Health Economics*, 12: 837–848.

Miller, D. K. and Homan, S. M. (1994) 'Determining transition probabilities: confusion and suggestions', *Medical Decision Making*, 14: 52–58.

O'Hagan, A., Stevenson, M. and Madan, J. S. (2005) 'Monte Carlo probabilistic sensitivity analysis for patient-level simulation models'. Sheffield Statistics Research Report 561/05. Sheffield, University of Sheffield.

Palmer, S., Sculpher, M., Philips, Z., Robinson, M., Ginnelly, L., Bakhai, A., *et al.* (2005) 'Management of non-ST-elevation acute coronary syndromes: how cost-effective are glycoprotein IIb/IIIa antagonists in the UK National Health Service?', *International Journal of Cardiology*, 100: 229–240.

Roderick, P., Davies, R., Raftery, J., Crabbe, D., Pearce, R., Patel, P., *et al.* (2003) 'Cost-effectiveness of population screening for *Helicobacter pylori* in preventing gastric cancer and peptic ulcer disease, using simulation', *Journal of Medical Screening*, 10: 148–156.

Stahl, J. E., Rattner, D., Wiklund, R., Lester, J., Beinfeld, M. and Gazelle, G. S. (2004) 'Reorganising the system of care surrounding laparoscpoic surgery: a cost-effectiveness analysis using discrete-event simulation', *Medical Decision Making*, 24: 461–471.

Stevenson, M. D., Oakley, J. and Chilcott, J. B. (2004) 'Gaussian process modelling in conjunction with individual patient simulation modelling: a case study describing the calculation of cost-effectiveness ratios for the treatment of established osteoporosis', *Medical Decision Making*, 24: 89–100.

UKPDS Study Group (1998) 'Intensive blood glucose control with sulphonylureas or insulin compared with conventional treatment and risk of complications in patients with type 2 diabetes', *Lancet*, 352: 837–853.

Chapter 4

Making decision models probabilistic

In this chapter, we describe how models can be made probabilistic in order to capture parameter uncertainty. In particular, we review in detail how analysts should choose distributions for parameters, arguing that the choice of distribution is far from arbitrary, and that there are in fact only a small number of candidate distributions for each type of parameter and that the method of estimation will usually determine the appropriate distributional choice. Before this review, however, consideration is given to the rationale for making decision models probabilistic, in particular the role of uncertainty in the decision process. There then follows a discussion of the different types of uncertainty, which focuses on the important distinction between variability, heterogeneity and uncertainty.

4.1. The role of probabilistic models

The purpose of probabilistic modelling is to reflect the uncertainty in the input parameters of the decision model and describe what this means for uncertainty over the outputs of interest: measures of cost, effect and cost-effectiveness (whether incremental cost-effectiveness ratios or net-benefit measures). However, there is a legitimate question as to what the role of uncertainty is in decision making at the societal level. In a seminal article, Arrow and Lind (1970) argued that governments should have a risk-bearing role when it comes to public investment decisions. The Arrow-Lind theorem would suggest therefore that decision makers might only be concerned with expected value decision making, and we might therefore question why uncertainty in cost-effectiveness modelling should concern us at all? We propose three main reasons why it is important to consider uncertainty, even if the concern of the decision maker is expected values. Firstly, most models involve combining input parameters in ways that are not only additive, but also multiplicative and as power functions, resulting in models that are nonlinear in those input parameters. Secondly, uncertainty over the results of an analysis implies the possibility of incorrect decision making which imposes a cost in terms of benefits forgone, such that there may be value of obtaining more information (thereby reducing uncertainty) even in a world where our only interest is in expected values. Finally, policy changes are rarely costless exercises and decision reversal may be problematic, such that there may exist value associated with delaying a decision that may be impossible, or problematic, to reverse. Each of these reasons is explored in more detail below, and we conclude the section with a discussion of potential biases if the estimation of expected value were the only interest in decision models.

4.1.1. Uncertainty and nonlinear models

Once we move beyond simple decision trees, which are linear in the input parameters, to Markov models and other more sophisticated models, the model structure essentially becomes nonlinear. This is due to the fact that the outputs of the model can be a multiplicative function of the input parameters. For example, even a very simple Markov model will involve multiplying the underlying transition probability parameters together to generate the Markov trace, which is an inherently nonlinear construct.

It is common, in statistics, to be reminded that, for a nonlinear transformation, $g(.)$, the following equality does not hold:

$$E\big[g(.)\big] \neq g\big(E[.]\big).$$

That is, the expectation of the transformation does not equal the transformation of the expectation (Rice 1995). The same is true of decision models as statistical models. We can consider our model a nonlinear transformation function (albeit a complex one). Our fundamental interest is in the expected value of the output parameters (costs, effects and cost-effectiveness), but we will not obtain this expectation by evaluating the model at the expected values of the input parameters. Instead, it will be necessary to specify input distributions for input parameters of the model and propagate this uncertainty through the model to obtain a distribution over the output parameters. It is then the expectation over the output parameters that represent the point estimate for the decision model.

For this reason, even if the decision maker is convinced that their only interest is in the expected value of the model, it is still necessary to consider uncertainty in the input parameters of a nonlinear model rather than simply employ the point estimates. Nevertheless, in all but the most nonlinear models, the difference between the expectation over the output of a probabilistic model and that model evaluated at the mean values of the input parameters, is likely to be modest, suggesting the bias in the latter approach is usually not a major concern.

4.1.2. **Value of information**

It is often wrongly assumed that a fundamental interest in making decisions on the basis of expected cost-effectiveness means that uncertainty is not relevant to the decision-making process. For example, in a provocatively titled article, Claxton (1999) proclaimed the 'irrelevance of inference', where he argued against the arbitrary use of 5 per cent error rates in standard medical tests of hypothesis. Unfortunately, some readers have interpreted the irrelevance of inference argument to mean that decisions should be taken only on the basis of the balance of probabilities, that is, that a greater than 50 per cent probability is sufficient justification for recommending a treatment option.In fact, Claxton argues for a much more rational approach to handling uncertainty that avoids arbitrary error rates. Uncertainty is argued to be costly in that there is always a risk that any decision made is the wrong one. Where incorrect decisions are made, then society will suffer a loss as a consequence. Therefore, in the decision theoretic approach (Pratt *et al.* 1995), value is ascribed to the reduction of uncertainty (or the creation of additional information) such that a decision may include the option to acquire more information.

Note that the decision theoretic approach acknowledges that information gathering entails a cost; therefore the decision to acquire more information involves balancing the costs of acquiring more information with its value, such that a decision to collect more information is not simply an exercise in delaying a decision. Value-of-information methods are described in detail in Chapter 7. For the purposes of this chapter, we simply note that the value-of-information approach has at its heart a well-specified probabilistic model that captures parameter uncertainty in such a way that uncertainty in the decision can be adequately reflected and presented to the decision maker.

4.1.3. **Option values and policy decisions**

Value-of-information methods implicitly assume that *current* decisions should be made on the basis of expected cost-effectiveness, but that where there is value in reducing uncertainty and collecting additional information, *future* decisions might change the expected value such that the current decision needs to be overturned. This notion of expected value decision making may not adequately reflect that policy changes are not costless, and more importantly, may be difficult or impossible to reverse. Palmer and Smith (2000) argue that the options approach to investment appraisal can offer insight into the handling of uncertainty and decision making in health technology assessment. They argue that most investment decisions exhibit the following characteristics:

- Future states of the world are *uncertain.*
- Investing resources is essentially *irreversible.*
- There is some discretion over investment *timing.*

Under these conditions, they argue that it would be optimal to adjust cost-effectiveness estimates in line with an options approach to valuing the 'option' to make a decision, assuming that as time progresses additional information will become available that may reduce some of the uncertainties inherent in the decision. The authors acknowledge the essentially passive nature of the emergence of additional information in the options literature and suggest that it would be optimal to integrate the options approach into the value-of-information approach discussed previously.

4.1.4. Potential for bias in decision models

In the three subsections above, we argue the case for why it is important for analysts to represent uncertainty in their decision models even if decision makers are only interested in expected values. An implicit assumption behind expected value decision making is that unbiased estimates of cost-effectiveness are available. Yet in some settings, such as in pharmaceutical company submissions to reimbursement agencies, there may be clear incentives that may encourage bias in decision models. For example, there are two bodies in the UK that consider cost-effectiveness evidence: the Scottish Medicines Consortium (SMC) in Scotland and the National Institute for Health and Clinical Excellence (NICE) in England and Wales. The SMC considers cost-effectiveness at the launch of products and invites submissions only from the manufacturers of products. NICE considers products later in the lifecycle of technologies, and commissions an independent appraisal of the technology from an academic group in addition to considering evidence from manufacturers. It is clear that there is a keen incentive for manufacturers to 'make a case' for their product, which could lead to potential bias in favour of their products.

If the only requirement to claim cost-effectiveness was a model that showed a point estimate of cost-effectiveness that falls into an acceptable range, then it is possible that combinations of parameter values could be chosen to generate the required result with no consideration of the underlying uncertainty. While the requirement to explicitly include a probabilistic assessment of uncertainty (as is now required by NICE (2004)) does not guarantee that models produced will be unbiased, direct consideration of uncertainty may make it slightly more difficult to manipulate analyses directly in favour of a treatment because of the clear and direct link to the evidence base.

4.2. **Variability, heterogeneity and uncertainty**

Having argued that it is important for analysts to incorporate uncertainty estimates for the parameters into their models, it is worth considering precisely the form of the uncertainty that is to be captured. Unfortunately, there exists much confusion surrounding concepts related to uncertainty in economic evaluation and it is often the case that the literature does not use terms consistently. In this section, we distinguish between variability (the differences that occur between patients by chance) and heterogeneity (differences that occur between patients that can be explained) from decision uncertainty – the fundamental quantity that we wish to capture from our decision models. We begin by considering the concepts of variability, heterogeneity and uncertainty. We then introduce an analogy with a simple regression model to explain each concept and argue that the concepts can equally be applied to a decision model.

4.2.1. **Variability**

When we consider patient outcomes, there will always be variation between different patients. For example, suppose a simple case series follows a group of severe asthmatics with the aim of estimating the proportion of patients that experience an exacerbation of their asthma in a 12-week period compared with those that did not. Suppose that of 20 patients followed, four experience an exacerbation within the 12-week period such that the estimated proportion is 0.2 or 20 per cent. If we consider the group to be homogeneous then we would consider that each patient has a 20 per cent chance of having an exacerbation over the follow-up period. However, each individual patient will either have an exacerbation or not, such that there will be variability between patients even if we know that the true probability of an exacerbation is 20 per cent. This variability between subjects has been referred to as *first order uncertainty* in some of the medical decision-making literature (Stinnett and Paltiel 1997), however it may be best to avoid such terminology as it is not employed in other disciplines.

4.2.2. **Heterogeneity**

While variability is defined above as the random chance that patients with the same underlying parameters will experience a different outcome, heterogeneity relates to differences between patients that can, in part, be explained. For example, as we can see from any standard life table, age and sex affect mortality rates – women have lower mortality than men (of the same age) and, beyond the age of 30, mortality increases approximately exponentially with age. Note that if we condition on age and sex, there will still be variability between individuals in terms of whether or not they will die over a specified period of, for example, 20 years. The distinction between heterogeneity and variability is important – we often seek to understand and model heterogeneity, as it is quite possible that policy decisions will vary between individuals with different characteristics. Heterogeneity is not a source of uncertainty as it relates to differences that can be explained. For example, mortality rates may vary by age and sex and, given age and sex, there may be uncertainty in the mortality rate. For a given individual, however, their age and sex will be known with certainty.

4.2.3. **Uncertainty**

In terms of the previous section, it is uncertainty that we are seeking to capture in our decision models, rather than variability or heterogeneity. It is worth differentiating two forms of uncertainty: parameter uncertainty and model (or structural) uncertainty. The first of these is internal to the model and the second is effectively external to the model.

To the extent that parameters of a given model are estimated, they will be subject to uncertainty as to their true value; this is known as parameter uncertainty. This type of uncertainty has sometimes been termed *second order uncertainty* to distinguish it from *first-order uncertainty* (or variability) as discussed above. An example would be the previously discussed estimate of the proportion of exacerbations. The estimated proportion was 20 per cent based on the observation of four events out of 20. We are concerned with the certainty of this estimate and we could employ standard statistical methods to represent uncertainty in our estimate. The standard approach is to recognize that the data informing the parameter estimate follow a binomial distribution and that the standard error of the proportion can be obtained from the binomial distribution:

$$se(\bar{p}) = \sqrt{\bar{p}(1-\bar{p})/n}$$

where $\bar{p}$ is the estimated proportion and n is the sample size. In the example above, where $\bar{p} = 0.2$ and $n = 20$, $se(\bar{p}) = 0.09$ and the 95% confidence interval (0.02–0.38) is obtained by taking 1.96 standard errors either side of the point estimate.

To understand the distinction between variability between patients and uncertainty in the estimate of the proportion, consider that instead of observing four events from 20, we had instead observed 400 events out of 2000. As the proportion is still 20 per cent, the variability between patients remains unchanged, however, the uncertainty in our estimate of the proportion is much reduced at $se(\bar{p}) = 0.009$ and associated 95% confidence interval (0.18–0.22).

It is not just parameter uncertainty that is important, however, we must also consider the importance of model (or structural) uncertainty. Model (or structural) uncertainty relates not to the parameters themselves, but to the assumptions imposed by the modelling framework. Any estimate of uncertainty based on propagating parameter uncertainty through the model will be conditional on the structural assumptions of the model and it is important to recognize that different assumptions could impact the estimated uncertainty.

4.2.4. An analogy with regression models

In the three previous subsections we distinguish between the concepts of variability, heterogeneity and (parameter/model) uncertainty. Part of the reason for confusion with these concepts in the literature is a lack of consistency in terminology. In this section, therefore, we offer an analogy with a standard regression model that should be applicable across a variety of disciplines. Consider the standard regression model:

$$Y = \alpha + \sum_{j=1}^{p} \beta_j X_j + \varepsilon$$

which relates a dependent variable Y to p independent variables $X_j, j = 1 \ldots p$. The intercept α and coefficients β are the parameters to the model and can be estimated by ordinary least squares. The error term is given by ε.

All of the concepts described above in relation to decision models can be given an analogous explanation in terms of the standard regression equation given above. The estimated value of Y represents the output parameter of the model, while the α and β values are the input parameters. The β coefficients represent heterogeneity in that different values of the covariates X (e.g. patient characteristics) will give different fitted values. Note that additional parameters are required to model the heterogeneity. Parameter uncertainty is given by the estimates of standard error for the α and β parameters of the model. Variability (or unexplained heterogeneity) is encapsulated by the error term of the model. Finally, note that the fitted values of the model and the uncertainty of the estimated parameters are conditional on the model itself. The model above assumes a simple additive relationship between the independent and dependent variables. We might also consider a multiplicative model, for example, by assuming that covariates relate to the log of the dependent variable. This would lead to a different set of estimated fitted values; the difference between the two estimates relates to model uncertainty (Draper 1995). Note that the focus of the remaining sections of the chapter is the characterization of parameter uncertainty. We return to representing model uncertainty in Chapter 5.

4.3. **Choosing distributions for parameters**

In this section we consider how to choose and fit distributions for parameters of decision models, under the assumption of a homogeneous sample of patients informing parameter estimation. The use of regression modelling to handle parameters that are a function of covariates is handled subsequently, including the use of survival analysis to estimate probabilities.

One criticism often levelled at probabilistic decision models is that the choice of distribution to reflect uncertainty in a given parameter is essentially arbitrary, which adds an additional layer of uncertainty that must itself be subjected to sensitivity analysis. In this section we argue that this is not the case. Rather, the type of parameter and its method of estimation will usually reveal a small number of (often similar) candidate distributions that should be used to represent uncertainty. These distributions will often reflect the standard distributional assumptions employed to estimate confidence intervals, as described in almost any introductory medical statistics text (Altman 1991; Armitage and Berry 1994). Indeed, we would argue that by following standard approaches to distributional assumptions whenever possible, the quality and credibility of the analysis will be enhanced. We begin by describing the use of the normal distribution, as this is effectively a candidate distribution for any parameter through the *central limit theorem*, and then go on to consider individual parameter types.

Note that although a formal Bayesian perspective could (and some would argue should) be adopted when fitting distributions to parameters, it is not the purpose of this chapter to review formal Bayesian methods. We therefore adopt a rather informal approach to fitting distributions to parameters based on the evidence available which will, in general, lead to very similar distributions to a formal Bayesian analysis with uninformative prior distributions. Excellent introductions to the formalities of the Bayesian approach can be found in the book by Gelman and colleagues (1995) and a specific primer on cost-effectiveness analysis by O'Hagan and Luce (2003).

4.3.1. **The normal distribution and the central limit theorem**

As was introduced in Chapter 1 and further discussed earlier in this chapter, the fundamental interest for the cost-effectiveness analyst is with expectations (mean values). In capturing parameter uncertainty in the estimation of the expected value of a parameter, we need to represent the sampling distribution of the mean. The *central limit theorem* is an important theorem in respect of the sampling distribution of the mean. The theorem essentially states that the sampling distribution of the mean will be normally distributed irrespective of the underlying distribution of the data with sufficient sample size. This has profound implications for our choice of distribution for any of our parameters in that the normal distribution is a candidate distribution for representing the uncertainty in any parameter of the model.

In deciding whether to use the normal distribution, the issue becomes one of whether the level of data informing the estimation of the parameter is of sufficient sample size to justify the normal assumption. Recall the previously introduced example of observing four exacerbation results out of 20, where it was argued that the data informing the estimation of the proportion was binomially distributed. In Fig. 4.1, the discrete binomial distribution for possible values of the proportion is shown as the grey bars. Overlaid is the normal distribution based on the estimated standard error of 0.09 and above the normal distribution is an I-bar representing the previously calculated 95% confidence interval (0.02–0.38).

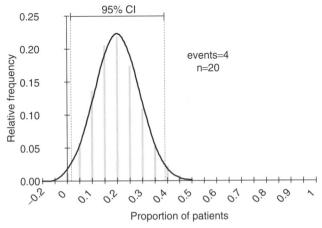

Fig. 4.1 Binomial distribution for estimated proportion based on four events out of 20 with normal distribution overlaid.

It is clear from Fig. 4.1 that the use of the normal distribution in this context is not appropriate as there would be a non-negligible probability of sampling an impossible value – in this case a probability below zero. Note that it would not be appropriate to simply discard impossible values in this context. If we were to use the normal distribution shown in Fig. 4.1, but discarded any value that was drawn that was less than zero, we would effectively be drawing from a truncated normal distribution. However, the problem is that the truncated normal distribution would no longer have the mean and variance that was originally chosen. We return to how the uncertainty in the estimation of the proportion in this example should be handled below.

4.3.2. Distributions for probability parameters

Probability parameters have an important constraint – all probabilities can only take values between the range of zero and one. Furthermore, probabilities of mutually exclusive events must sum to one. When selecting distributions for probability parameters, it is therefore important that the probability parameters continue to obey these rules, even once the random variation is introduced. Exactly how the distribution of probability parameters is determined depends on the method of estimation. Below we deal with probabilities estimated from a binomial proportion and from the multinomial equivalent in a univariate context.

Beta distribution for binomial data

The earlier example illustrated in Fig. 4.1 related to a proportion of 0.2 based on four events out of 20. This proportion is the natural estimate of the probability of an event. However, we have already seen that a normal approximation is not appropriate for these data – so how should the uncertainty in the estimated probability be represented? The solution to the problem comes from a standard result in Bayesian statistics – the beta distribution enjoys a special relationship with binomial data, such that if a prior is specified as a beta distribution, then that distribution can be updated when binomial data are observed to give a beta distributed posterior distribution (Gelman *et al.* 1995). This relationship between the beta and binomial distribution is termed *conjugacy*, with the beta distribution described as conjugate to binomial data. For our purposes, the technicalities of the Bayesian solution are not required (although the interested reader is directed to the technical appendix). Rather, it is simply that the beta distribution is a natural choice for representing uncertainty in a probability parameter where the data informing that parameter are binomial.

The beta distribution is constrained on the interval 0–1 and is characterized by two parameters, α and β. When data are binomially distributed, fitting the

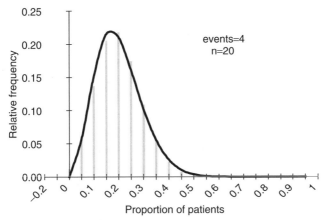

Fig. 4.2 Binomial distribution for estimated proportion based on four events out of 20 with a beta(4,16) distribution overlaid.

beta distribution turns out to be extremely straightforward. If the data are represented by a number of events of interest r, observed from a given sample size n, the proportion of events to the total sample gives the point estimate of the probability. Uncertainty in this probability can be represented by a beta (α,β) distribution, simply by setting $\alpha = r$ and $\beta = n-r$. Figure 4.2 shows the result of fitting a beta(4,16) distribution to the data of the previous example. It is clear that the beta distribution fits the data very well and exhibits the desired properties of not allowing probabilities outside of the logical constraints.

Dirichlet distribution for multinomial data

Instead of having binomial data, it is often common for the data to be divided into a number of categories; that is, the data are multinomial. Recall the example of the HIV/AIDS model developed in Chapter 2 and with the transition matrix reported in Table 2.2. The original article reported that the transitions were estimated from a cohort of patients from the Chelsea and Westminster Hospital in the UK (Chancellor *et al.* 1997). The counts from which the probabilities were estimated were reported in Table 2.5 (as part of Exercise 2.5), where each row of the table represents the data from which transition probabilities can be estimated. It should be clear, for example, that the probability of transition from AIDS (State C) to death (State D) is estimated by $1312/1749 = 0.75$ and that the uncertainty in this estimate can be represented by a beta(1312, 437) distribution – but what about the transitions from States A and B? The data informing these transitions are naturally multinomial – with four and three categories respectively. The Dirichlet distribution, which is the multivariate generalization of the beta distribution with parameters equal to the number of categories in the multinomial distribution, can be used to represent, in a probabilistic fashion, the transition probabilities for transiting among polytomous categories (or model states). Mathematical details for the fitting of Dirichlet distribution are given in the technical appendix, but note that the fitting of the Dirichlet distribution is just as easy as that of the beta distribution, with parameters having the interpretation of 'effective sample sizes' (Gelman *et al.* 1995). Thus the uncertainty in the transition probabilities from State A of the model are simply represented by a Dirichlet(1251, 350, 116, 17) distribution and from State B by a Dirichlet(731, 512, 15). The ease of fitting is the primary reason for employing the Dirichlet distribution, as a series of conditional beta distributions will generate exactly the same results (see appendix). Further details on the use of the Dirichlet distribution, including a discussion of the use of priors to counter potential zero observations in the transition matrix can be found in the paper by Briggs and colleagues (2003).

Fitting beta distributions by method of moments

In the two previous subsections, we emphasize just how easy it is to fit beta (Dirichlet) distributions to binomial (multinomial) data when counts of the event of interest plus its complement are available. However, it is not always the case that such counts are available or even appropriate. For example, when fitting beta distributions to secondary data or meta-analysis results, it may only be the mean/proportion and standard error/variance that are reported. If this is the case then it is still possible to fit the beta distribution using an approach known as method of moments. For $\theta \sim \text{beta}(\alpha,\beta)$ the moments of the beta distribution are given by:

$$E[\theta] = \frac{\alpha}{\alpha + \beta}$$

$$\text{var}[\theta] = \frac{\alpha\beta}{(\alpha + \beta)^2 (\alpha + \beta + 1)}.$$

If the sample moments $\bar{\mu}$ and s^2 are known then we simply equate the sample moments to the distribution moments:

$$\bar{\mu} = \frac{\alpha}{\alpha + \beta}$$

$$s^2 = \frac{\alpha\beta}{(\alpha + \beta)^2 (\alpha + \beta + 1)}$$

and rearrange to give the unknown parameters as a function of the known sample mean and variance:

$$(\alpha + \beta) = \frac{\bar{\mu}(1-\bar{\mu})}{s^2} - 1$$
$$\alpha = \bar{\mu}(\alpha + \beta).$$

For example, if instead of knowing that four events out of 20 were observed, only the proportion of 0.2 and the binomial estimate of standard error of 0.09 were reported, it would still be possible to fit the beta distribution parameters. From the equation above, we calculate $\alpha = 0.2^2 \cdot 0.8 / 0.09^2 - 0.2 = 3.75$ and we can then calculate:

$$\beta = \alpha \cdot \frac{(1-\mu)}{\mu}$$
$$= 3.75 \cdot 0.8 / 0.2$$
$$= 15$$

and, therefore, fit a beta(3.75,15). Note that the slight difference in the fitted distribution comes about due to the rounding errors introduced by using figures from a published source.

4.3.3. Distributions for relative risk parameters

Relative risk parameters are one of the most common parameter types used to incorporate the effect of treatment into models. In order to understand the appropriate distribution to choose and how to fit it, it is worth looking at the background of how a relative risk is calculated and how the confidence interval is constructed. A generic two-by-two table is shown in Table 4.1 with n representing the total observations and a, b, c and d representing the cell counts.

The relative risk is defined:

$$RR = \frac{a}{a+c} \bigg/ \frac{b}{b+d}$$
$$= \frac{a}{a+c} \cdot \frac{b+d}{b}.$$

Table 4.1 Standard two-by-two table for estimating relative risk

	Treatment group	Control group	Total
Event present	a	b	a + b
Event absent	c	d	c + d
Total	a + c	b + d	n

As the relative risk is made up of ratios, it is natural to take the log to give:

$$\ln(RR) = \ln(a) - \ln(a + c) + \ln(b + d) - \ln(b).$$

The standard error of this expression is given by:

$$se\left[\ln(RR)\right] = \sqrt{\frac{1}{a} - \frac{1}{a+c} + \frac{1}{b} - \frac{1}{b+d}}$$

which can be used to calculate the confidence interval on the log scale in the usual manner. To obtain the confidence interval on the relative risk scale, the log scale confidence limits are simply exponentiated.

Knowing that confidence limits for the relative risk parameters are calculated on the log scale suggests that the appropriate distributional assumption is lognormal. To fit the distribution to reported data is simply a case of deconstructing the calculated confidence internal. Continuing with the HIV/AIDS model example – the authors of the original paper employ a relative risk estimate of 0.51 with a quoted 95% confidence interval of 0.365–0.710 (Chancellor *et al.* 1997), which they apply to the baseline transition probabilities in the Markov model. Taking the natural logs of the point and interval estimates generates the following log scale estimates: −0.675 (−1.008, − 0.342). Dividing the range through by 2 × 1.96 recovers the estimate of log scale standard error:

$$se\left[\ln(RR)\right] = \frac{-0.342 - -1.008}{2 \times 1.96} = 0.173.$$

Now we simply take a random draw from a N(−0.675, 0.170) distribution and exponentiate the result.

The approach described above is based on replicating the standard approach of reporting relative risks in the medical literature. Note, however, that the mean of a lognormal distribution calculated in this way will not return the original relative risk estimate. For example, the quoted relative risk in the equation above is 0.509, but the mean of a lognormal distribution with mean of −0.675 and standard error of 0.170 (both on the natural log scale) will give an expected value on the relative risk scale of 0.517. This simply reflects the fact that the standard reporting of relative risk is for the modal value on the relative risk scale rather than the mean. As is clear from this example, the difference between the mode and the mean on the relative risk scale is rather small. We return to the issue of estimating costs on the log scale later in this chapter, where the difference between the mean and mode on the original scale is of much greater importance.

4.3.4. **Distributions for costs**

Just as our choice of distribution for probability data was based upon the range of the data, so it should be noted that cost data are constrained to be non-negative and are made up of counts of resource use weighted by unit costs. Count data are often represented by the Poisson distribution (which is discrete) in standard statistical methods. The gamma distribution also enjoys a special relationship with Poisson data in Bayesian statistics (the gamma is conjugate to the Poisson, which means that posterior parameter distributions for Poisson data are often characterized by gamma distributions). This suggests that a gamma distribution, which is constrained on the interval 0 to positive infinity, might be used to represent uncertainty in cost parameters.

Another alternative, which is often employed in regression analyses, is the lognormal distribution. Both the lognormal and the gamma distributions can be highly skewed to reflect the skew often found in cost data. Here we illustrate fitting a gamma distribution to represent uncertainty in a skewed cost parameter. The use of the lognormal distribution for costs is illustrated later in this chapter as part of a discussion of regression methods.

To fit a gamma distribution to cost data we can again make use of the method of moments approach. The gamma distribution is parameterized as $\text{gamma}(\alpha,\beta)$ in Excel and the expectation and variance of the distribution can be expressed as functions of these parameters as given below:

$$\theta \sim \text{gamma}(\alpha,\beta)$$
$$E[\theta] = \alpha\beta$$
$$\text{var}[\theta] = \alpha\beta^2.$$

A note of caution is that some software packages (e.g. TreeAge DATA) parameterize the gamma distribution with the reciprocal of the beta parameter (i.e. $\beta' = 1/\beta$) and so care must be taken about which particular form is used.

The approach is again to take the observed sample mean and variance and set these equal to the corresponding expressions for mean and variance of the distribution:

$$\bar{\mu} = \alpha\beta, \qquad s^2 = \alpha\beta^2.$$

It is then simply a case of rearranging the expressions and solving the two equations for the two unknowns simultaneously:

$$\alpha = \frac{\bar{\mu}^2}{s^2}, \qquad \beta = \frac{s^2}{\bar{\mu}}.$$

Again taking as an example a parameter from the HIV/AIDS model, consider the direct medical costs associated with the AIDS state of the model, which is reported in the original article as £6948 (Chancellor *et al.* 1997). Unfortunately, although this estimate seems to have been taken from a patient-level cost data set, no standard error was reported. For the purposes of this example, suppose that the standard error is the same value as the mean. We can estimate the parameters of the gamma distribution from the equations above as $\alpha = 6948/6948 = 1$ and $\beta = 6948^2/6948 = 6948$, hence we fit a gamma(1,6948).

4.3.5. **Distributions for utilities**

Utility parameters are clearly important in health economic evaluation, but represent slightly unusual parameters in terms of their range. The theoretical constraints on utility parameters in terms of their construction are infinity at the lower end (representing the worse possible health state) and 1 at the upper end (representing perfect health).

A pragmatic approach, often employed when health state utilities are far from zero, is to use a beta distribution. However, this is not appropriate for states close to death where values less than one are possible.

A simple transformation of $D = 1 - U$, such that D is a utility decrement or a disutility provides the solution. This utility decrement is now constrained on the interval 0 to positive infinity and the previous methods of fitting a lognormal or gamma distribution can be applied.

4.3.6. **Is there a role for triangular distributions?**

It is common to see probabilistic analyses presented with parameter distributions represented by the triangular distribution. Triangular distributions are typically represented by three parameters: a minimum, a maximum and a mode. The distribution itself is simply a triangle with unit area with the apex at the mode and the probability going down to zero at the minimum and maximum values. The mean and variance of the triangular distribution are given by:

$$\text{mean} = \frac{1}{3}\left(\text{min} + \text{mode} + \text{max}\right)$$

$$\text{var} = \frac{1}{18}\left(\text{min}^2 + \text{mode}^2 + \text{max}^2 - \text{min}\cdot\text{mode} - \text{min}\cdot\text{max} - \text{mode}\cdot\text{max}\right).$$

The apparent popularity of the triangular distribution may come from the fact that it is simple to fit, requiring only three points to be specified. However, as a representation of uncertainty, it often leaves a lot to be desired.

The central point of the triangular distribution is the mode, not the mean. Therefore, if the modal value is not the central point between the minimum and maximum values, the distribution is non-symmetric and the mean will not equal the mode. The distribution itself has three points of discontinuity at each of the minimum, mode and maximum, which is unlikely to represent our beliefs about the uncertainty in a parameter (is there really absolutely zero chance of being below the minimum?) Finally, minima and maxima are poor statistics in the sense that the range of variation measured tends to increase with sample size as there is more of a chance of observing an extreme value. It is generally considered desirable for the variance of a parameter distribution to diminish when we have greater information on that parameter.

Consider how we might fit a triangular distribution to the simple proportion parameter where four events are observed out of 20. We certainly might make the modal value 0.2, but how would we set the minimum and maximum values? Setting them equal to the logical constraints of 0 and 1 for the parameter is not advisable – by doing so, the mean of the distribution would become $1.2/3 = 0.4$ which is not what we would want to use. We could try setting the minimum and maximum as 0 and 1 then solve for the mode, giving a mean of 0.2 – but it should be clear that there is no such result for this example. A method of moments type approach, based on a symmetric distribution would result in a minimum value of less than zero. The point of this example is to emphasize that while the triangular distribution is apparently simple, and might therefore be considered an appealing choice of distribution, the lack of a link to the statistical nature of the estimation process hampers rather than helps the choice of parameters of the distribution.

4.4. Drawing values from the chosen distribution

Having considered which distributions may be appropriate for representing uncertainty in different types of parameter distribution, we now consider the mechanics of how we can draw random values from these distributions.

Most software packages include some form of random number generator (RNG) that will give a pseudo random number on the interval 0–1. As all values within the interval are equally likely, this RNG gives a uniform distribution. This uniform distribution forms the building block of random sampling.

4.4.1. The uniform distribution and the cumulative distribution function

We need a way of mapping a random draw from a uniform distribution to a random draw from a distribution that we specify. To do this, we need a little background on distribution functions.

The distribution that we wish to draw from is a probability density function (pdf) which defines (for a continuous function) the probability that a variable falls within a particular interval by means of the area under the curve. The characteristic feature of a pdf is that the total area under the curve integrates to 1.

The cumulative distribution function (cdf) defines the area under the pdf to a given point. Therefore the cdf is constrained on the interval 0–1. It is the cdf that can provide the appropriate mapping from a uniform distribution to the corresponding pdf.

To see how this mapping occurs, consider Fig. 4.3. The top right-hand panel shows the cdf for the standard normal distribution (i.e. N(0,1)). Note that the vertical axis runs from zero to one.

Now consider a random draw from the uniform distribution (top left panel of the figure) from this 0–1 interval. By reading across from the vertical axis to the cdf curve and down to the horizontal axis, we map a random draw from the uniform distribution to a random draw from the N(0,1) distribution. Repeating this process a large number of times will generate an empirical picture of the N(0,1) pdf shown in the bottom right panel of the figure.

Of note is that in using the mapping process above we are effectively using the *inverse* of the cdf function. Usually, specifying a value of the variable in a

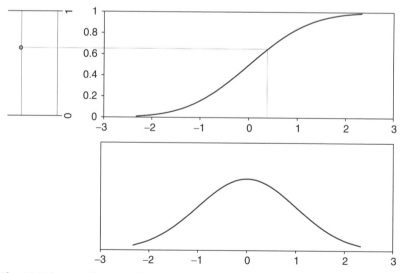

Fig. 4.3 Using a uniform random number generator and the inverse cumulative distribution function to generate a random draw from the corresponding probability density function.

cdf function returns the integrated probability density to that point. Instead, we specify the integrated probability and get the value. In Excel, the NORMDIST(x,0,1,1) gives the integrated probability p from the standard normal. The inverse cdf is NORMINV(p,0,1) = x, which can be made probabilistic by replacing p with the RAND() function.

4.4.2. **Correlating parameters**

A common criticism of probabilistic sensitivity analysis is that parameters are assumed to be independent. However, it is important to realize that while this is commonly what happens in applied analyses, it is possible to correlate parameters if the covariance structure between them is known. Rather, the problem is more that analysts usually have no data on the covariance structure and so choose not to model covariance (in either direction).

One example where we clearly do know the covariance relationship of parameters is in a regression framework, where we have access to the variance–covariance matrix. In this situation, we can employ a technique known as Cholesky decomposition to provide correlated draws from a multivariate normal distribution. Obtaining correlations between other distributional forms is not straightforward; instead the approach taken (in common with many other statistical procedures) is to search for a scale on which multivariate normality is reasonable.

Cholesky decomposition for multivariate normal distributions

The starting point for the Cholesky decomposition method is the variance–covariance matrix, such as would be obtained from a standard regression, call this matrix **V**. The Cholesky decomposition of matrix **V** is a lower triangular matrix (a matrix where all cells above the leading diagonal are zero), call this matrix **T**, such that **T** multiplied by its transpose gives the covariance matrix, **V**. In this sense, we can think of **T** as being like the square root of the covariance matrix.

Once matrix **T** has been calculated, it is straightforward to use it to generate a vector of correlated variables (call this vector **x**). We start by generating a vector (**z**) of independent standard normal variates and apply the formula: **x** = **y** + **Tz**, where **y** is the vector of parameter mean values.

It can sometimes be difficult to understand conceptually how Cholesky decomposition works. Indeed, the best way to understand Cholesky decomposition is to see it working in practice by doing a small example by hand and working through the algebra. In this simple example we assume just two parameters to be correlated. The starting point is to write down the general form for a Cholesky decomposition matrix, **T** and to multiply **T** by its transpose to give a 2 × 2 matrix. This matrix can then be set equal to the variance–covariance matrix:

$$\begin{pmatrix} a & 0 \\ b & c \end{pmatrix}\begin{pmatrix} a & b \\ 0 & c \end{pmatrix} = \begin{pmatrix} a^2 & ab \\ ab & b^2+c^2 \end{pmatrix} = \begin{pmatrix} \mathrm{var}(x_1) & \mathrm{cov}(x_1,x_2) \\ \rho se(x_1)se(x_2) & \mathrm{var}(x_2) \end{pmatrix}.$$

For a known variance–covariance matrix, it is straightforward to solve for the unknown a, b and c components of the Cholesky decomposition matrix in terms of the known variance and covariance:

$$\begin{pmatrix} a & 0 \\ b & c \end{pmatrix} = \begin{pmatrix} \sqrt{\mathrm{var}(x_1)} & 0 \\ \mathrm{cov}(x_1,x_2)/a & \sqrt{\mathrm{var}(x_2)-b^2} \end{pmatrix} = \begin{pmatrix} se(x_1) & 0 \\ \rho\cdot se(x_2) & \sqrt{1-\rho^2}\cdot se(x_2) \end{pmatrix}.$$

To generate correlated random variables we go back to the original Cholesky equation of $\mathbf{x} = \mathbf{y} + \mathbf{Tz}$:

$$\begin{pmatrix} x_1 \\ x_2 \end{pmatrix} = \begin{pmatrix} \mu_1 \\ \mu_2 \end{pmatrix} + \begin{pmatrix} a & 0 \\ b & c \end{pmatrix}\begin{pmatrix} z_1 \\ z_2 \end{pmatrix}.$$

Multiplying this expression out gives

$$\begin{pmatrix} x_1 \\ x_2 \end{pmatrix} = \begin{pmatrix} \mu_1+a\cdot z_1 \\ \mu_2+b\cdot z_1+c\cdot z_2 \end{pmatrix}$$

and then substituting in the definitions of a, b and c we have defined previously gives:

$$\begin{pmatrix} x_1 \\ x_2 \end{pmatrix} = \begin{pmatrix} \mu_1+se(x_1)\cdot z_1 \\ \mu_2+\rho\cdot se(x_2)\cdot z_1+\sqrt{1-\rho^2}\cdot se(x_2)\cdot z_2 \end{pmatrix}$$

from which it is apparent how the procedure is working. For example, the first random variable will clearly have the mean and standard error required. The second random variable will also have a mean and standard error given by the associated parameter's mean and standard error. The correlation is introduced through the shared component of variance z_1 in proportion to the overall correlation.

Generating rank order correlation

As mentioned above, while Cholesky decomposition can be employed to correlate multivariate normal parameters, the correlation of other types of distribution are less straightforward. A practical solution is to correlate the ranks of random draws from distributions rather than focus on the (Pearson) correlation coefficient. This can be achieved by setting up a matrix of correlations to be achieved and then using this correlation matrix to draw random parameters from the multivariate standard normal distribution using the Cholesky decomposition method as described above. Having generated these random draws which have the required correlation structure, they can be back transformed to a uniform distribution using the standard normal distribution. This vector of draws from the uniform distribution has rank order correlation between the parameters given by the original correlation matrix. The individual elements can then be combined with the desired inverse cumulative density functions to generate rank order correlations between non-normal distributions.

4.5. Regression models for handling heterogeneity

Previously, our concern was with choosing distributions when fitting parameters to a single group of homogeneous patients. However, it is rare that patients are truly homogeneous and it is common to use regression methods to explore heterogeneity between patients. In the sections below a number of regression models are introduced. All share the same basic structure, being based around a linear predictor, but the form and scale of the regressions differ according to the nature of the data.

4.5.1. Logistic regression to estimate probabilities from binomial data

In a paper looking at the cost-effectiveness of ACE-inhibitors for the treatment of stable coronary disease, Briggs *et al.* (2006) employed a regression model to calculate the probability of death conditional on having had a primary clinical endpoint from the clinical trial (a combined endpoint of myocardial infarction, cardiac arrest and cardiovascular death). The data to which the model was fitted were binomial – from a total of 1091 primary clinical endpoints, 406 (37 per cent) were fatal. The fitted model was a standard logistic regression model of the form:

$$\ln\left(\frac{\pi}{1-\pi}\right) = \alpha + \sum_{j=1}^{p} \beta_j X_j$$

where π represents the probability of death, the term on the left is the log-odds of death, and where the covariates are assumed to have an additive effect on the log-odds scale. The results are shown in Table 4.2, which suggests that age, cholesterol level and a history of a previous myocardial infarction all increase the odds of an event being fatal, given that the primary clinical endpoint has occurred.

Table 4.2 Logistic regression for the probability of having a fatal event given that a primary clinical endpoint has occurred

Covariate	Coefficient	Standard error	Odds ratio	95% Confidence interval
Age	0.040	0.007	1.040	1.026–1.054
Cholesterol	0.187	0.057	1.206	1.079–1.347
Previous myocardial infarction	0.467	0.150	1.596	1.188–2.142
Intercept	−4.373	0.598		

It should be clear from the form of the logistic regression model above that exponentiating both sides will generate a multiplicative model of the odds, such that the exponentiated coefficients from Table 4.2 are odds ratios. These are shown in the fourth column of the table together with their corresponding 95% confidence intervals. In order to generate the probability of a fatal event it is necessary to go one step further and rearrange the equation above to give the following expression for the estimated probability:

$$\hat{\pi} = \frac{\exp\left\{\alpha + \sum_{j=1}^{p}\beta_j X_j\right\}}{1 + \exp\left\{\alpha + \sum_{j=1}^{p}\beta_j X_j\right\}}.$$

So, for example, to estimate the probability of a fatal event for a 65-year-old, with a cholesterol level of 6 mmol/l and a history of previous myocardial infarction, we first estimate the linear predictor (LP) as

$$LP = -4.373 + 65 \times 0.040 + 6 \times 0.187 + 0.467$$
$$= -0.184$$

and then substitute this estimate into the equation above to give the probability as:

$$\hat{\pi} = \frac{\exp\left\{-0.184\right\}}{1 + \exp\left\{-0.184\right\}}$$
$$= 0.454$$

that is, an elevated risk compared with the overall mean of 37 per cent chance of a fatal event.

Although the probability of a fatal event is the parameter of interest in the above model, it could be considered as an endogenous parameter, being fully determined by other, exogenous, parameters – the coefficients from the regression results. If we want to represent uncertainty around the probability parameter there are two broad approaches that could be used. Firstly, the Cholesky decomposition method could be employed as described previously, under the assumption that the coefficients in Table 4.2 follow a multivariate normal distribution.

The covariance–correlation matrix for the logistic regression model above is shown in Table 4.3. The leading diagonal shows the variances and above the leading diagonal, the covariances between the coefficients are shown. As the covariance matrix is symmetric, the cells below the leading diagonal show the correlation coefficients. It is clear from these coefficients that there is considerable correlation between the estimated intercept term and the other parameters, and moderate correlation between the age and cholesterol coefficient parameters.

An alternative, but equivalent, method for estimating the uncertainty in the probability is to note that the general (matrix) formula for the variance of a linear predictor (LP) is given by $\mathrm{var}(LP_0) = \mathbf{X}_0^T \mathbf{V} \mathbf{X}_0$, where $\mathbf{X}_0$ is the column vector of covariates for a given individual patient (and $\mathbf{X}_0^T$ a row vector being its transpose) and $\mathbf{V}$ representing the variance–covariance matrix for the coefficient parameters. For our example:

$$\mathrm{var}(LP_0) = (65 \quad 6 \quad 1 \quad 1) \begin{pmatrix} .000047 & .000075 & .000047 & -.003421 \\ .000075 & .003201 & -.000402 & -.022327 \\ .000047 & -.000402 & .022592 & -.017710 \\ -.003421 & -.022327 & -.017710 & .357748 \end{pmatrix} \begin{pmatrix} 65 \\ 6 \\ 1 \\ 1 \end{pmatrix}$$

$$= 0.0059$$

Table 4.3 Covariance (*correlation*) matrix for the logistic regression model of Table 4.2. Leading diagonal shows the variances and above the leading diagonal the covariance between parameters. Below the leading diagonal, the correlation between parameters is shown

	Age	Cholesterol	Previous myocardial infarction	Intercept
Age	0.000047	0.000075	0.000047	−0.003421
Cholesterol	*0.19*	0.003201	−0.000402	−0.022327
Previous myocardial infarction	*0.05*	*−0.05*	0.022592	−0.01771
Intercept	*−0.83*	*−0.66*	*−0.20*	0.357748

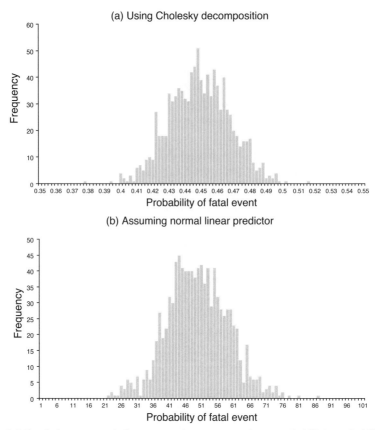

Fig. 4.4 Simulating two equivalent approaches to generating a probabilistic probability parameter from a logistic regression model.

which can be used as the variance in a normal distribution with mean equal to the point estimate of the linear predictor. Random draws from this distribution can be used to estimate the uncertainty in the probability once the inverse logistic transformation is applied.

The equivalence of the two approaches can be seen in Fig. 4.4 which shows the histogram of a Monte Carlo simulation for the probability of a fatal event using each approach. Although there are some slight differences apparent in the histograms, this results from random chance. The mean values (standard deviations) of the Cholesky and normal linear predictor approaches from the simulations were 0.448 (0.019) and 0.446 (0.019), respectively.

4.5.2. **Survival analysis to estimate probabilities from time-to-event data**

In Chapter 3, the use of standard survival analysis methods for the estimation of transition probabilities in Markov models is discussed. In particular, the use of the Weibull model for the hazard of failure is highlighted. Recall that the Weibull model is a two parameter proportional hazards model, with shape parameter γ, and a scale parameter λ. Also recall from Fig. 3.2 how different values of γ lead to very different shapes for the underlying hazard function. The formulae for the Weibull distribution and the corresponding hazard and survivor functions are given below:

$$f(t) = \lambda \gamma t^{\gamma-1} \exp\left\{-\lambda t^\gamma\right\}$$
$$h(t) = \lambda \gamma t^{\gamma-1}$$
$$S(t) = \exp\left\{-\lambda t^\gamma\right\}.$$

Our concern in this section is to illustrate how heterogeneity between patients can be modelled in the context of a parametric survival analysis. This is usually achieved by assuming that covariates act (in proportionate fashion) on the scale parameter, but that the shape parameter remains the same for all patients.[1] In algebraic terms we specify:

$$\ln \lambda = \alpha + \sum_{j=1}^{p} \beta_j X_{ij}$$

such that the value of the lambda is constructed from the exponential of the linear predictor from a regression.

As an example, consider the Weibull regression of late prosthesis failure from the total hip replacement model reported in Table 4.4 (Briggs *et al.* 2004). The second column gives the estimated coefficients from the Weibull model on the log scale with the log scale standard error in column three. Exponentiating the estimated coefficients give the hazard ratios in the case of the covariates, the baseline hazard in the case of the intercept and the value of the shape parameter. The intercept (or log of the baseline hazard) relates to

---

[1] It is possible to parameterise the shape parameter in terms of covariates. However, this makes the representation much more complex (for example, by parameterizing the shape parameter of the Weibull model it would no longer be a proportional hazards model). In practice, such models are rarely reported and we are unaware of any application in the health economic evaluation field that have yet used such models.

Table 4.4 Weibull survival model for the hazard of late prosthesis failure

Covariate	Coefficient	Standard error	exp(coefficient)	95% Confidence interval
Spectron prosthesis	−1.34	0.383	0.26	0.12–0.55
Years over age 40	−0.04	0.005	0.96	0.95–0.97
Male	0.77	0.109	2.16	1.74–2.67
Intercept	−5.49	0.208	0.0041	0.0027–0.0062
Gamma parameter	0.37	0.047	1.45	1.32– 1.60

a 40-year-old woman given the standard (Charnley) prosthesis. Exponentiating the linear predictor gives the value of λ for the Weibull model. For example, the baseline hazard is the λ value for a 40-year-old woman with a Charnley prosthesis at the point of the primary replacement (i.e. time point zero). The value of λ for a 60-year-old man who has been given the Spectron prosthesis is calculated as:

$$\lambda = \exp\left\{-5.49 + (60 - 40) \times -0.04 + 0.77 - 1.34\right\}$$
$$= 0.0011.$$

The gamma parameter of the Weibull distribution is also presented in Table 4.4 and is also estimated on the log scale. The exponentiated coefficient is significantly greater than one, but also less than two, suggesting that the hazard function increases over time, but at a decreasing rate.

Once the shape and scale parameters are estimated, the calculation of the transition probability (as a function of the patient characteristics) proceeds just as described in Chapter 3. The question becomes how to incorporate uncertainty into the estimation of the transition probability. The covariance–correlation matrix for the Weibull model of Table 4.4 is shown in Table 4.5 with variances of the estimated coefficients on the leading diagonal, covariance above the leading diagonal and correlation coefficients below.

In the previous section, in the context of logistic regression, it was argued that there were two approaches to incorporating uncertainty in the estimated probability – either to use the Cholesky decomposition of the covariance matrix or to estimate the variance of the linear predictor from the covariance matrix directly. Note, however, that the latter approach is not appropriate for survival models with more than a single parameter. If we were to estimate λ and its associated uncertainty from the linear predictor directly and then employ that parameter along with the estimated value of γ together with its

Table 4.5 Covariance (*correlation*) matrix for Weibull model of Table 4.5

	Spectron	Years over 40	Male	Intercept	Gamma
Spectron	0.146369	−0.000111	0.000184	−0.000642	0.000259
Years over 40	*−0.06*	0.000027	0.000033	−7.83E-04	2.80E-08
Male	*0.00*	*0.06*	0.011895	−0.007247	0.000051
Intercept	*−0.01*	*−0.72*	*−0.32*	0.043219	−0.005691
Gamma	*0.01*	*0.00*	*0.01*	*−0.58*	0.002252

uncertainty in a Weibull model to estimate a transition probability, we would be neglecting the correlation between the two parameters. Such a case is illustrated in the upper part of Fig. 4.5 where the left-hand panel shows the independent random sampling of the λ and γ parameters (assuming normality on the log scale), and the right-hand panel shows the associated transition probability estimates over time including estimated 95% confidence intervals.

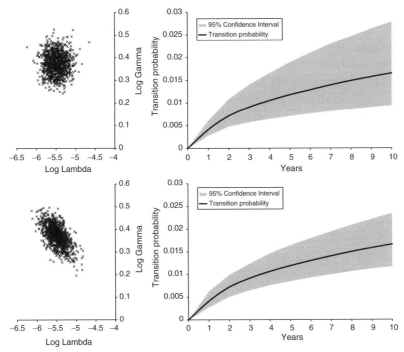

Fig. 4.5 The impact of correlating parameters in a Weibull survival regression on the uncertainty of estimated transition probabilities The top panel shows the consequences of failing to account for correlation between the parameters. Appropriate correlation is shown in the bottom panel.

Table 4.6 Ordinary least squares regression of age on cost of primary care over four month period of the UKPDS

Covariate	Coefficient	Standard error	95% Confidence interval
Age	0.83	0.24	0.36–1.30
Constant	22.40	15.08	–7.17–51.97

Contrast this with the lower part of Fig. 4.5, which shows the equivalent results but where Cholesky decomposition is employed to ensure that the λ and γ parameters are appropriately correlated on the log scale (assuming joint normality). Notice that by including the appropriate correlation, the uncertainty in the estimated transition probabilities is substantially reduced.

4.5.3. Regression models to estimate cost/utility data

As with considering univariate parameters for cost or utility decrements/ disutilities (see earlier), the normal distribution is a candidate when using regression methods to adjust for heterogeneity (through the *central limit theorem*). However, both costs and utility decrements can exhibit substantial skewness which may cause concern for the validity of the normal approximation. Consider the ordinary least squares regression model reported in Table 4.6, showing the relationship between age and primary care costs over a 4-month period in patients participating in the UK Prospective Diabetes Study (1998).

The results suggest that each year of age increases the 4-month cost of primary care by 83 pence. If these results were to be used in a probabilistic model, then it would be possible to estimate cost from the above regression using either Cholesky decomposition or the variance of linear predictor method described above. However, examination of standard regression diagnostic plots presented in Fig. 4.6 suggests reasons to be cautious of the normal assumption. The residual distribution is clearly highly skewed and the residual versus fitted plot suggests possible heteroskedacticity.

A common approach to handling skewness is to consider fitting a regression model to the natural log of cost, in the case of the UK Prospective Diabetes Study (UKPDS) data, the model would be:

$$\ln(C_i) = \alpha + \beta \times age_i + \varepsilon_i. \tag{4.1}$$

This model is presented in Table 4.7, with the corresponding regression diagnostics (on the log scale) in Fig. 4.7.

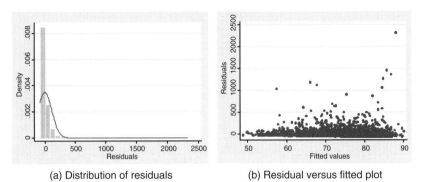

(a) Distribution of residuals   (b) Residual versus fitted plot

Fig. 4.6 Regression diagnostics for the ordinary least squares on 4-month primary care cost.

This model suggests that each year of age increases cost by 0.7 per cent of cost, rather by a fixed amount. The regression diagnostics for this model look much better behaved on the log scale (see Fig. 4.7). However, in any probabilistic model it will be necessary to estimate costs on the original scale, but retransformation back from the log scale is not straightforward due to the nonlinear nature of the transformation. For example, the estimate of expected cost on the original scale is not obtained by exponentiating the linear predictor from eqn 4.1 above:

$$E[C_0] \neq \exp\{\bar{\alpha} + \bar{\beta} \times \text{age}_0\}.$$

Rather, it turns out that a smearing correction must be applied (Duan 1983; Manning 1998), which in the case of the log transformation of costs corresponds to a factor equal to the mean of the exponentiated log scale residuals:

$$E[C_0] = \exp\{\alpha + \beta \times \text{age}_0\} \times \frac{1}{n}\sum_{i=1}^{n} \exp\{\varepsilon_i\}.$$

This added factor complicates the adaptation of log transformed regression models as the smearing factor becomes an additional parameter to the model. An alternative approach to modelling costs is to use a generalized linear model

Table 4.7 Ordinary least squares regression of age on the natural log of primary care cost over a 4-month period in the UKPDS

Covariate	Coefficient	Standard error	95% Confidence interval
Age	0.007	0.002	0.003–0.011
Constant	3.315	0.137	3.047–3.583

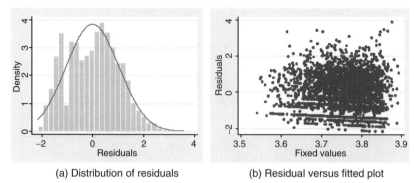

(a) Distribution of residuals   (b) Residual versus fitted plot

Fig. 4.7 Regression diagnostics for the ordinary least squares on the natural log of 4-month primary care cost.

(GLM) where a distribution for the underlying data is assumed together with a scale for the linear predictor. GLMs have gained in popularity for modelling costs as they model the expectation of the cost directly. For the UKPDS example, a GLM can be written as:

$$g(E[C_i]) = \alpha + \beta \times age_i \tag{4.2}$$

where the function $g(.)$ is known as the link function. This link function specifies the scale of measurement on which the covariates are assumed to act in linear fashion. In the case of the log link, it should be clear from eqn 4.2 that the expected cost is obtained by simple exponentiation of the linear predictor. In Table 4.8, a GLM is presented for the UKPDS example assuming a gamma distribution for the cost data and a log link. The coefficients are therefore estimated on the log scale and are similar to those reported in Table 4.7.

In contrast to the results of the log transformed cost data, however, the back transformation to the raw cost scale is straightforward. For example, the expected primary care cost for a 60-year-old would be estimated as £73.26, which is calculated by $\exp\{3.634 + 60 \times 0.011\}$.

Table 4.8 Generalized linear model regression of age on primary care cost over a 4-month period in the UKPDS

Covariate	Coefficient	Standard error	95% Confidence interval
Age	0.011	0.002	0.005–0.017
Constant	3.634	0.137	3.259–4.010

4.5.4. A note on the use of GLMs for probabilistic analysis

However, care needs to be taken when using a GLM with a nonlinear link function as part of a probabilistic model. Examination of the covariance matrix reveals the covariance between the age coefficient and the constant term in the regression model is -0.000577. For the example of a 60-year-old, the linear predictor is $4.294 = 3.634 + 60 \times 0.011$ and its variance is estimated as $0.033 = 0.0137^2 + (60 \times 0.002)^2 + 2 \times 60 \;\; 0.002 \times -0.000577$. Therefore, it would be natural in a probabilistic model to assume a lognormal distribution for mean cost by drawing from a normal distribution with mean 4.294 and variance 0.033 before exponentiating the result. However, it is important to recognize that the mean of a lognormal distribution is given by the exponent of the log mean plus half the log variance. Therefore, if the expectation of the probabilistic distribution is to correspond to the mean of the cost from a log link GLM, it is necessary to adjust the log mean by taking away half the log variance. For the example of the 60-year-old, by sampling from the normal distribution with mean $4.294 - 0.033 / 2$ and variance 0.033 the resulting lognormal cost distribution will have the desired mean of £73.26. (In this example the correction factor is unimportant as the mean of the lognormal distribution with mean 4.294 and variance 0.033 on the log scale is only £74.48, however, for much higher costs or more skewed/uncertain parameter estimates the difference could be much more substantial.)

4.6. Summary

The purpose of this chapter has been to argue that the choice of probability distribution to represent uncertainty in decision analytic models is far from arbitrary. As the focus of the analysis is on estimating expected values of parameters, the normal distribution is always a candidate distribution due to the *central limit theorem*. However, this theorem is based on asymptotics and decision models are often constructed with parameters that are informed by very little data. In such situations, the choice of distribution should be informed by the logical constraints on the parameter and the form of the data/estimation process. Although other distributions, such as the triangular distribution, have proved a popular choice in the past, we argue against the use of these distributions on the basis that they bear little relationship to the sampling distribution of the mean of sampled data. As an *aide memoir*, Table 4.9, provides a summary of the types of parameters commonly encountered in health economic models, logical constraints on those parameters and candidate distributions for the parameters based on the data/estimation process.

Table 4.9 Summary of common parameter types and candidate distributions for univariate estimation

Parameter (logical constraints)	Form of data and method of estimation	Candidate distribution	Excel command
Probability $(0 \leq \pi \leq 1)$	Binomial: estimated proportion	Beta(α,β), $\alpha,\beta > 0$	BETAINV(.)
	Multinomial: estimated proportions	Dirichlet$(\alpha_1, \ldots \alpha_k)$, $\alpha_k > 0\ \forall_k$	None (see appendix)
	Time to event: survival analysis	Lognormal(lm,lv), lm, lv > 0	EXP(NORMINV(.))
Relative risk $(\theta > 0)$	Binomial: ratio of estimated proportions	Lognormal(lm,lv), lm, lv > 0	EXP(NORMINV(.))
Cost $(\theta \geq 0)$	Weighted sum of resource counts: mean	Gamma(α,β), $\alpha,\beta > 0$	GAMMAINV(.)
		Lognormal(lm,lv), lm, lv > 0	EXP(NORMINV(.))
Utility decrement/ Disutility $(\theta \geq 0)$	Continuous non-zero: mean	Gamma(α,β), $\alpha,\beta > 0$	GAMMAINV(.)
		Lognormal(lm,lv), lm, lv > 0	EXP(NORMINV(.))
All parameters	Any distribution of data	Normal(μ, σ^2), $\sigma^2 > 0$	NORMINV(.)

In addition, we have attempted to illustrate the appropriate handling of heterogeneity through regression methods and the importance of including parameter correlations into any probabilistic model. We have argued that the distinction between variability, uncertainty and heterogeneity is important, and although variability is not as important for decision making per se as it is in the environmental literature (Thompson and Graham 1996; Thompson 2002), the separation of variability and heterogeneity from uncertainty underlies better decision making, as we discuss in the remaining chapters.

4.7. **Exercise: making the HIV/AIDS model probabilistic**

4.7.1. **Overview**

The aim of this exercise is to demonstrate how the deterministic HIV/AIDS model from Exercise 2.5 can be made probabilistic by fitting distributions to parameters. Emphasis is on choosing the correct distribution for different types of parameters and in particular on the use of the Dirichlet distribution for generating a probabilistic transition matrix, where constant transitions are appropriate.

The step-by-step guide below will take you through a number of stages of making the model probabilistic:

1. Using a lognormal distribution for relative risk.
2. Using a gamma distribution for cost.
3. Using a beta distribution for the transition from AIDS to death.
4. Using a Dirichlet distribution for the transition matrix.

A template for the exercise, 'Exercise 4.7 – template.xls', is available, based on the solution to Exercise 2.5 adapted to allow additional information to be entered.

4.7.2. **Step-by-step guide**

On opening the exercise template spreadsheet, take a moment to examine the changes from the spreadsheet solution to Exercise 2.5. In particular, you will see that the parameter list is now labelled 'live' and that cell C3 allows switching between a probabilistic model and generating a deterministic point estimate (from columns C and D respectively). Make sure the switch for the probabilistic model is set to zero, so that the deterministic column D appears in the live cells (column B). The general task in this exercise is to complete the probabilistic column C so that when the switch in C3 is set to 1 the model becomes fully probabilistic.

1. Using a lognormal distribution for relative risk

In the original Chancellor *et al.* (1997) article, the quoted relative risk was 0.509 with 95% confidence interval 0.365–0.710. Use this information to calculate the appropriate log mean and log standard error in cells F35 and G35. In cell C35, take a random draw from the normal distribution (with the mean and standard error you just calculated) and exponentiate to give the lognormally distributed relative risk.

2. Using a gamma distribution for cost

In rows 21 through 26 the direct medical and community care costs associated with each state of the model are listed. Unfortunately, little information was given in the original article about the variance of costs (despite the fact that mean costs were derived from a patient level dataset). A simple assumption has therefore been made that the standard error of the costs is equal to the mean. Hence, the entry in column E is simply the same as that in column D. Using the information in columns D and E and the formula given in the section 'Distributions for costs', use the method of moments approach to solve for the parameters of the gamma distribution and enter these values in columns F and G. Now generate a random draw from the gamma distribution using these parameters and enter in column C.

3. Using a beta distribution for the transition from AIDS to death

As mentioned in the presentation, a beta distribution can be used for a dichotomous decision probability and is straightforward to fit using the counts already given in columns F and G of the number of events (deaths) observed and the complement (total – deaths). Therefore, in cell C17 generate a random draw from the beta distribution using the values in cells F17 and G17 as parameters. Note that the value in cell C16 must, by definition, be 1 minus the value of C16 (in other words do not sample from two independent beta distributions as probabilities must sum to one).

4. Using a Dirichlet distribution for polytomous transitions

This chapter previously detailed how the Dirichlet distribution is the multinomial equivalent of the beta distribution that can be used when more than two transitions are possible. Unfortunately, Excel does not include the Dirichlet directly, therefore it must be constructed. This is relatively straightforward, but does require an extra step.

    i. Start with the three-way transition from State B to remaining in State B, or moving to State C (AIDS), or moving to State D (death), as detailed in rows 13–15. The method is to normalize a draw from three independent single parameter gamma distributions, where the single parameter is the number of events. Note the single parameter gamma distribution is simply the usual two parameter distribution with the second (beta) parameter set to 1. Therefore in cells E13 to E15, enter a random draw from a gamma distribution with the alpha parameter set to the value in column F and the beta parameter equal to 1 (do not be alarmed if Excel returns an error – see below).

ii. Now there is a problem in Excel: it solves the gamma distribution by iteration and when the value of alpha is very high (over about 300) it will often fail to find a solution (what you see is a '!NUM' error message) due to the iterative procedure Excel uses to solve the gamma function. However, for high values of the alpha parameter in the single gamma function, the resulting distribution is not at all skewed and tends toward the normal distribution. Therein lays the solution to the problem. For high values of alpha, we substitute a random draw from the normal distribution with the equivalent mean and variance of the gamma distribution. Recall that the variance of the gamma distribution (from the presentation) is alpha*beta^2. Therefore, as beta = 1 for the single parameter gamma, the variance is simply alpha. Either do this by hand in cells E13 and E14, or else set up an IF statement to choose the correct distribution automatically.

iii. Once, you have valid numbers in cells E13 to E15, the corresponding probability in column C is calculated as the corresponding draw in column E divided by the sum of E13:E15. This ensures that all probabilities are in the range 0–1 and that the three probabilities sum to 1. Enter the appropriate formula in cells C13 to C15. Congratulations! You have just constructed your first Dirichlet distribution.

iv. Now repeat the three steps above, but this time for the four probabilities associated with State A in rows 9–12.

You now have a fully probabilistic model. If you switch cell C3 to equal 1 and then turn to the *<Analysis>* worksheet you should find that a single draw from the model is made each time you press <F9>.

4.8. Exercise: making the total hip replacement model probabilistic

4.8.1. Overview

The aim of this exercise is to demonstrate how the deterministic total hip replacement (THR) model from Exercise 3.5 can be made probabilistic by fitting distributions to parameters. Emphasis is on choosing the correct distribution for different types of parameters and on correlating parameters using the Cholesky decomposition of a variance–covariance matrix.

The step-by-step guide below will take you through a number of stages of making the model probabilistic:

1. Setting up the <Parameters> worksheet for probabilistic analysis.

2. Fitting beta distributions to (constant) probability parameters.

3. Fitting gamma distributions to cost parameters.

4. Fitting beta distributions to utility parameters.

5. Correlating parameters by Cholesky decomposition and application to the regression model for prosthesis survival.

A template for the exercise, '*Exercise 4.8 – template.xls*', is available, based on the solution to Exercise 3.5.

4.8.2. **Step-by-step guide**

1. Setting up the *<Parameters>* worksheet for probabilistic analysis

On opening the file you will find that the parameters screen has changed and the point estimates of the parameters that you used in the previous exercise have been moved to column D (labelled 'deterministic'). This means that the model no longer works, as all the 'live' parameter cells are currently blank. Take a moment to familiarize yourself with the new layout of this worksheet. In particular, note the addition of cell D3 that, in conjunction with the new layout, will enable us to 'switch' between a deterministic and probabilistic version of the model.

    i. Firstly, note that not all parameters have been labelled as potential candidates for the probabilistic analysis: patient characteristics (age and sex), discount rates and prosthesis costs have all been coloured black indicating they are to be left deterministic. Before starting on the exercise, ensure that you are totally happy with why these parameters will not form part of the probabilistic analysis.

    ii. The first step is to use an IF(…) statement to determine what appears in column B dependent on the value in cell D3. The idea is to be able to switch between deterministic values (column D) and probabilistic values (column C) easily. Note that cell B25 should be excluded from this (in addition to the deterministic parameters referred to above). You will recall that the lambda parameter from the regression is endogenous to the model – therefore, it will by definition be deterministic or probabilistic depending on the nature of the other parameters that make it up. Note that just as B25 is exponentiated, so must B26 be (to get a lognormal distribution). To do this, you can exponentiate the whole of the IF(…) statement.

iii. Now enter 0 in cell D3 and verify that the results on the *<Analysis>* worksheet and match the results from Exercise 3-5. When cell D3 is switched to the value 1, column B should be populated with empty values.

Now that the restructuring of the *<Parameters>* worksheet is complete, the rest of the exercise is concerned with fitting probabilistic values to the parameters in column C such that when cell D3 is set to 1, the model becomes fully probabilistic.

2. Fitting beta distributions to (constant) probability parameters

The following information has been provided to you concerning operative mortality rates following primary surgery:

> The hospital records of a sample of 100 patients receiving a primary THR were examined retrospectively. Of these patients, two patients died either during or immediately following the procedure. The operative mortality for the procedure is therefore estimated to be 2 per cent.

i. Use this information to specify the parameters (alpha and beta in columns G and H) of a beta distribution for the probability of operative mortality during primary surgery.

ii. Use the BETAINV(…) function in cell C16 to generate a random draw from this distribution.

iii. As no information is available on operative mortality following a revision procedure, use the same distribution again for this parameter (row 17).

The following information has been provided to you concerning revision procedures among patients already having had a revision operation.

> The hospital records of a sample of 100 patients having experienced a revision procedure to replace a failed primary THR were reviewed at one year. During this time, four patients had undergone a further revision procedure.

iv. Use this information to fit a constant transition probability for the annual re-revision rate parameter (row 18).

You should now have three probabilistic parameters in C16:C18 that should automatically generate a new value from the specified distribution when you hit the <F9> key.

v. Use the formula for the moments of a beta distribution from the section on 'Distributions for probability parameters' in order to specify the mean and standard error (columns D and E) for these distributions.

vi. How do these compare with the mean values and standard errors that would have been calculated from these data using standard methods?

Hint: in order to answer this question you need to recall that the binomial standard error is estimated from the formula: $se = \sqrt{p(1-p)/n}$.

3. Fitting gamma distributions to cost parameters

As the costs of prostheses are handled deterministically, the cost of the primary procedure is ignored (as it is assumed to be the same in each arm). In addition, there is assumed to be no cost of monitoring successful procedures, so there is only really one probabilistic cost to specify for the model – the cost of the revision procedure.

You are given the following information regarding the cost of revising a failed primary THR:

> A number of units involved in THR were reviewed and the mean cost of a revision procedure was found to be £5294 with a standard error of £1487.

  i. Add the value for the standard error into the spreadsheet (cell E33).

  ii. Use the method of moments approach described in the presentation to calculate the parameters (cells G33 and H33) of a gamma distribution that has the corresponding mean and standard error.

  iii. Use the GAMMAINV(...) function in cell C33 to generate a random draw from this distribution.

An alternative approach would have been to fit a normal distribution for this parameter – do you think this would be valid in this case?

4. Fitting beta distributions to utility parameters

As was indicated in Section 4.3.2, there are two methods to fitting the beta distribution. Here the second approach is taken using method of moments to fit beta distributions to the utility data.

You are given the following information on utilities for patients experiencing different states of the model:

The following information has been provided to you concerning operative mortality rates following primary surgery:

> A study was instigated to explore the utility weights subjects placed on different outcomes of THR related to the states of the Markov model – the following results were calculated in terms of mean (standard error) by state:
> Successful primary – 0.85 (0.03)
> Successful revision – 0.75 (0.04)
> Revision – 0.3 (0.03)

  i. Enter the standard errors into the worksheet (E41:E43).

  ii. Obtain the beta parameters corresponding to these mean values and standard errors by method of moments.

  iii. Use the BETAINV(...) function in cells C41:C43 to generate random draws from these distributions

5. Application of Cholesky to the regression model for prosthesis survival

We now implement the Cholesky decomposition matrix method in the model. Look at the *<Hazard function>* worksheet, which gives the results of a regression analysis for the hazard ratio. You have used these results before when constructing the deterministic model, but now we have added the covariance matrix for the parameters (together with the correlation matrix, which is a little easier to interpret). It should be clear that, while some parameters do not have a strong relationship, there are strong relationships within this set of parameters – particularly between the regression constant and the other parameters.

i. Note that the covariance matrix you have been given is a 5×5 matrix. You have been given a lower triangular Cholesky decomposition of the covariance matrix in cells C26:G31. Take a few moments to understand how this was obtained (you may want to refer back to the section on correlating parameters).

ii. In cells C36:C40, use the NORMINV(…) function to generate five random draws from the standard normal distribution.

iii. In cells E36:E40, enter the solution of the **Tz** matrix calculation, that is the Cholesky decomposition matrix multiplied by the vector of standard normal variates.

iv. Now add the estimated mean values from the regression to **Tz** and enter into cells G36:G40.

v. You have now created a vector of five multivariate normal parameters that are correlated according to the estimated covariance matrix. The final task is to go to the *<Parameters>* worksheet and link the probabilistic cells C22:C24 and C26:C7 to the relevant cell of the vector you have just created.

vi. Although not essential to the working of the parameters worksheet, for completeness you should add in the standard errors and distribution for the parameters you have just entered.

vii. Remember that we have been working on the log hazard scale for the Weibull regression. We need to make sure that the model parameters are exponentiated. This should already have been done for the endogenous lambda parameter in cell B25 (check that this is the case). The gamma parameter and the parameter relating to the relative risk of the new prosthesis should also be exponentiated. Note this can either be done by exponentiating the IF(…) function in column B or by separately exponentiating the deterministic and probabilistic values in columns C and D.

viii. Congratulations! The model should now be probabilistic. Verify this by switching cell D3 to the value 1 and examining the *<Analysis>* worksheet.

4.9. **Technical appendix**

Probabilities for dichotomous branches in decision trees are often estimated from data where r events of interest are observed from n observations. Such data are characterized by the two parameter binomial distribution, $\text{Bin}(\pi, n)$, where π is the probability of an event and n is the number of observations. If the number of events r follows the binomial distribution then:

$$p(r) = \binom{n}{r} \pi^r (1-\pi)^{n-r}.$$

In a probabilistic model, the challenge is to specify a (continuous) distribution for the probability π of the event. In a Bayesian framework, this is most naturally achieved by specifying a prior distribution for π from the beta distribution $\text{beta}(\alpha, \beta)$, as this continuous distribution is conjugate to the binomial distribution and is bounded on the 0–1 interval (as probabilities must be). The prior belief of a probability of an event can be specified by the beta distribution:

$$p(\pi) = \frac{\Gamma(\alpha+\beta)}{\Gamma(\alpha)\Gamma(\beta)} \pi^{\alpha-1} (1-\pi)^{\beta-1}$$

where $\Gamma(u)$ represents the single parameter gamma function.

Bayes' theorem states that the posterior probability of a parameter is proportional to the prior probability of the parameter times the data likelihood. Applying Bayes' theorem to the example of binomial data with a beta prior gives:

$$p(\pi) \propto \pi^r (1-\pi)^{n-r} \pi^{\alpha-1} (1-\pi)^{\beta-1}$$
$$\propto \pi^{\alpha+r-1} (1-\pi)^{\beta+n-r-1}$$

which identifies the posterior distribution as $\text{beta}(\alpha + r, \beta + n - r)$. In other words, in order to generate a continuous distribution for the probability of an event that is bounded on the 0–1 interval, it is necessary only to add the observed number of events and non-events, respectively, to the two parameters of the beta distribution representing prior beliefs and to use these quantities as the updated parameters of the (posterior) beta distribution. Where the prior distribution is formulated to be minimally informative, as with the beta(1,1) (which gives a uniform distribution over the 0–1 interval), the data will dominate that prior. Note that in the text, the technicalities of the Bayes approach were omitted such that the beta distribution was fitted directly to the data.

4.9.1. The polytomous case

Where data occur naturally across $k > 2$ categories, the data are said to follow the multinomial distribution, given by:

$$r \sim \text{multin}\left(n; \pi_1, \pi_2, \ldots, \pi_k\right)$$

$$p(r) = \binom{n}{r_1 \, r_2 \ldots r_k} \pi_1^{r_1} \pi_2^{r_2} \ldots \pi_k^{r_k}$$

for

$$r_j = 0, 1, 2, \ldots n; \quad \sum_{j=1}^{k} r_j = n.$$

It is now natural to formulate the decision problem with multiple branches and consider the distribution of the probabilities π_1, π_2, ..., π_k for each of the individual branches. This is achieved using the Dirichlet distribution, which is the multivariate generalization of the beta distribution and is given by:

$$\pi \sim \text{Dirichlet}\left(\alpha_1, \alpha_2, \ldots, \alpha_k\right)$$

$$p(\pi) = \frac{\Gamma\left(\alpha_1 + \ldots + \alpha_k\right)}{\Gamma(\alpha_1) \ldots \Gamma(\alpha_k)} \pi_1^{\alpha_1 - 1} \ldots \pi_k^{\alpha_k - 1}$$

where

$$\alpha_1, \ldots, \alpha_k > 0; \quad \sum_{j=1}^{k} \pi_j = 1.$$

The application of Bayes' theorem gives the following derivation for the posterior distribution of the probabilities:

$$p(\pi) \propto \pi_1^{\alpha_1 - 1} \ldots \pi_k^{\alpha_k - 1} \pi_1^{r_1} \ldots \pi_k^{r_k}$$

$$\propto \pi_1^{\alpha_1 + r_1 - 1} \ldots \pi_k^{\alpha_k + r - 1}$$

which identifies the posterior as Dirichlet $(\alpha_1 + r_1, \ldots, \alpha + r_k)$. Specifying a minimally informative prior, such as Dirichlet $(1, \ldots, 1)$ means that the data dominate the prior.

Note that for $k = 2$ categories, the Dirichlet is exactly equivalent to the beta distribution.

4.9.2. Sampling from the Dirichlet distribution

In this chapter, we have emphasized the convenience of the Dirichlet distribution in modelling uncertainty when parameters are estimated from multinomial data. However, sampling from the Dirichlet distribution is less straightforward as it is not commonly represented in standard software packages. One exception to this is the WinBUGS software (Spiegelhalter *et al.* 1998), designed for Bayesian analysis and freely available from http://www.mrc-bsu.cam.ac.uk/bugs/welcome.shtml. This software was originally designed to allow Bayesian analysis for nonconjugate prior distributions; however, as the Dirichlet and multinomial distributions are directly available within the package, sampling from the appropriate Dirichlet distribution is especially easy in WinBUGS.

For other software packages that do not include a direct representation of the Dirichlet distribution there are two approaches to generating a Dirichlet distribution (Gelman *et al.* 1995).

1. Normalized sum of independent gamma variables

Draw variables $x_1, x_2, \ldots x_k$ from independent gamma distributions with shape parameters $\alpha_1, \alpha_2, \ldots \alpha_k$ and a common scale parameter:

$$x_j \sim Gamma(\alpha_j, \beta).$$

Then the required probabilities are simply:

$$\pi_j = \frac{\alpha_j}{\sum_{j=1}^{k} \alpha_j}.$$

Equivalently, the x_j can be drawn from a chi-squared distribution with $2\alpha_j$ degrees of freedom.

2. Series of conditional beta distributions

First π_1 is drawn from a beta $(\alpha_1, \sum_{j=2}^{k} \alpha_j)$. Next, for each π_j in turn, $j = 2 \ldots k-1$, draw φ_j from a beta $(\alpha_j, \sum_{i=j+1}^{k} \alpha_i)$, and then set $\pi_j = (1 - \sum_{i=1}^{j-1} \pi_i)\varphi_j$. Finally, set $\pi_k = 1 - \sum_{i=1}^{k-1} \pi_i$.

It is this method that corresponds to the decomposition of a multi-branch node into a series of conditional dichotomous nodes. However, it should be clear from the derivations above that if the data are multinomial, this approach is far less convenient computationally.

References

Altman, D. G. (1991) *Practical statistics for medical research.* London, Chapman and Hall.

Armitage, P. and Berry, G. (1994) *Statistical methods in medical research*, 3rd edn. Oxford, Blackwell Scientific Publications.

Arrow, K. J. and Lind, R. C. (1970) 'Uncertainty and the evaluation of public investment decisions', *American Economic Review*, 60: 364–378.

Briggs, A. H., Ades, A. E. and Price, M. J. (2003) 'Probabilistic sensitivity analysis for decision trees with multiple branches: use of the Dirichlet distribution in a Bayesian framework', *Medical Decision Making*, 23: 341–350.

Briggs, A., Sculpher, M., Dawson, J., Fitzpatrick, R., Murray, D. and Malchau, H. (2004) 'The use of probabilistic decision models in technology assessment: the case of total hip replacement', *Applied Health Economics and Health Policy*, 3: 78–89.

Briggs, A. H., Mihaylova, B., Sculpher, M., Hall, A., Wolstenholme, J., Simoons, M., Ferrari, R., Remme, W. J., Bertrand, M. and Fox, K. (2006) 'The cost-effectiveness of perindopril in reducing cardiovascular events in patients with stable coronary artery disease using data from the EUROPA Study', *Heart* 92(Suppl 2): A36.

Chancellor, J. V., Hill, A. M., Sabin, C. A., Simpson, K. N. and Youle, M. (1997) 'Modelling the cost effectiveness of lamivudine/zidovudine combination therapy in HIV infection', *PharmacoEconomics*, 12: 54–66.

Claxton, K. (1999) 'The irrelevance of inference: a decision-making approach to the stochastic evaluation of health care technologies', *Journal of Health Economics*, 18: 341–364.

Draper, D. (1995) 'Assessment and propagation of model uncertainty', *Journal of the Royal Statistical Society, Series B*, 57: 45–97.

Duan, N. (1983) 'Smearing estimate: a nonparametric retransformation method', *Journal of the American Statistical Association*, 78: 605–610.

Gelman, A., Carlin, J. B., Stern, H. S. and Rubin, D. B. (1995) *Bayesian data analysis.* London, Chapman and Hall.

Manning, W. G. (1998) 'The logged dependent variable, heteroscedasticity, and the retransformation problem', *Journal of Health Economics* 17: 283–295.

National Institute for Clinical Excellence (NICE) (2004) *Guide to the methods of technology assessment.* London, NICE.

O'Hagan, A. and Luce, B. (2003) *A primer on Bayesian statistics in health economics and outcomes research.* Bethesda, MD, MedTap International.

Palmer, S. and Smith, P. C. (2000) 'Incorporating option values into the economic evaluation of health care technologies', *Journal of Health Economics*, 19: 755–766.

Pratt, J. W., Raiffa, H. and Schlaifer, R. (1995) *Introduction to statistical decision theory.* Cambridge, MA, MIT Press.

Rice, J. A. (1995) *Mathematical statistics and data analysis*, 2nd edn. Belmont, Duxbury Press.

Spiegelhalter, D. J., Thomas, A. and Best, N. (1998) *WinBUGS [1.3].* MRC Biostatistics Unit, University of Cambridge.

Stinnett, A. A. and Paltiel, A. D. (1997) 'Estimating CE ratios under second-order uncertainty: the mean ratio versus the ratio of means', *Medical Decision Making*, 17: 483–489.

Thompson, K. M. (2002) 'Variability and uncertainty meet risk management and risk communication', *Risk Analysis*, 22: 647–654.

Thompson, K. M. and Graham, J. D. (1996) 'Going beyond the single number: using probabilistic assessment to improve risk management', *Human and Ecological Risk Assessment*, 2: 1008–1034.

UK Prospective Diabetes Study (UKPDS) Group', (1998) 'Intensive blood-glucose control with sulphonylureas or insulin compared with conventional treatment and risk of complications in patients with type 2 diabetes (UKPDS 33). *Lancet*, 352: 837–853.

Chapter 5

Analysing and presenting simulation output from probabilistic models

The aim of this chapter is to explore exactly how probabilistic models, with all parameters being represented by their respective distributions, should be handled in terms of producing, analysing and then presenting the results of the probabilistic analysis. The chapter starts by looking at how to analyse and present large numbers of Monte Carlo simulation results of the output parameters of interest for the straightforward comparison of two alternative treatments. We then turn to the issue of calculating the sensitivity of the overall results to individual parameter values using standard analysis of covariance (ANCOVA) methods. These methods are illustrated using the AIDS/HIV model that was developed in the previous chapters based on the work by Chancellor *et al.* (1997). The cost-effectiveness acceptability curve (CEAC) is introduced and the advantages over the standard presentation of interval estimates of uncertainty are outlined.

The next section deals with the use of multiple cost-effectiveness acceptability curves to represent uncertainty and distinguishes the use of multiple curves in two very different situations. In the first, multiple acceptability curves are used to reflect the same treatment choice between alternative treatments in the presence of heterogeneity. In the second, multiple curves are employed to represent mutually exclusive treatment options. The final two sections present worked case studies of probabilistic modelling which highlight a number of features of probabilistic modelling, but serve to illustrate the two multiple curve situations in particular. The first example relates to estimating heterogeneity in cost-effectiveness analysis of the use of an ACE inhibitor in stable coronary heart disease for patients at different levels of cardiovascular risk (Briggs *et al.* 2006); and the second relates to the use of different management strategies for erosive oesophagitis (Goeree *et al.* 1999; Briggs *et al.* 2002a).

5.1. **Analysing simulation results: two treatment alternatives**

In this section we review the standard approaches to decision making in cost-effectiveness using the graphical cost-effectiveness plane, going on to consider how we present information under conditions of uncertainty, including an illustration of how to write macros in Excel to record simulation results. The use of interval estimates for cost-effectiveness is illustrated and we argue for the use of CEACs as a more general solution to the problem of presenting uncertainty in cost-effectiveness analysis. We complete the section by introducing the net-benefit statistic and showing how it can be used to generate acceptability curves.

5.1.1. **The cost-effectiveness plane**

The cost-effectiveness plane (Black 1990) is presented in Fig. 5.1 and shows the difference (treatment minus control) in effectiveness (ΔE) per patient against the difference in cost (ΔC) per patient. Plotting the effectiveness difference on the horizontal axis has the advantage that the slope of the line joining any point on the plane to the origin is equal to the incremental cost-effectiveness ratio (ICER) = $\Delta C/\Delta E$, the statistic of interest in cost-effectiveness studies. The plane can be defined as four separate quadrants that are labelled using the points of the compass to minimize confusion that can arise from alternative numbering schemes.

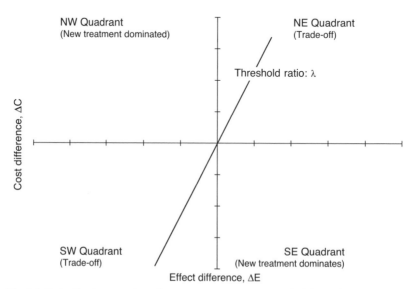

Fig. 5.1 Cost-effectiveness plane for new treatment compared with existing treatment.

If we consider the ideal circumstance of knowing the position of an intervention on the cost-effectiveness plane with no uncertainty, then a number of eventualities can arise. A new treatment is said to 'dominate' control, being less costly and more effective if it is located in the SE quadrant and vice versa – control dominates treatment if it is located in the NW quadrant. In these two circumstances it is clearly appropriate to implement the least costly and most effective (or dominant) treatment and no recourse to cost-effectiveness ratios is required. However, far more common is for one treatment to be more effective than the other, but also more costly. In such circumstances, a decision must be made as to whether the additional health benefits of the more effective treatment are worth the additional cost. If the ICER of the new therapy ($\Delta C/\Delta E$) – the slope of a straight line from the origin that passes through the (ΔE, ΔC) coordinate – is less than the acceptable 'threshold ratio' of the decision maker (representing the willingness-to-pay for a unit of health gain) then the treatment should be adopted.

Of course, the above discussion assumes that we know with certainty the cost, effect and cost-effectiveness of an intervention, such that the appropriate decision is clear. In practice, the outputs of our probabilistic models give us the distribution over incremental cost, incremental effect and the joint cost-effect distribution. For example, Fig. 5.2 shows 1000 Monte Carlo simulations

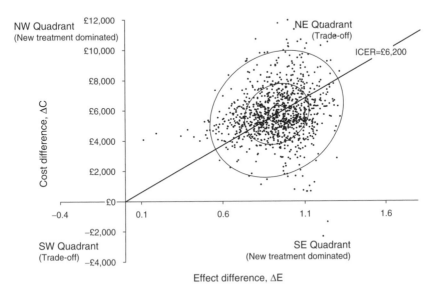

Fig. 5.2 Estimated joint cost-effectiveness density for the HIV/AIDS model plotted on the cost-effectiveness plane. Ellipses assume multivariate normality for the joint density with the same covariance structure as the simulations and cover 5%, 50% and 95% of the estimated joint density on the cost-effectiveness plane.

of the output of the AIDS/HIV model together with the elliptical joint density estimates assuming multivariate normality with the same variance–covariance as the simulations.

The presentation of the simulated joint density in Fig. 5.2 requires that the probabilistic output of our probabilistic models is recorded. As this is a straight forward repetitive process, it can be easily achieved in Excel using simple programs known as 'macros'. Box 5.1 outlines a simple approach to macro writing in Excel using the 'record' feature of the software.

Box 5.1: Example code for visual basic macro to record simulation results

The idea of writing macros can sound rather intimidating, particularly as macros are effectively written in the Visual Basic programming language. The macros themselves are stored in the 'Visual Basic Editor' which is separate from the main workbook (although all programming is saved as part of the workbook). Fortunately, to program macros, you need to know very little visual basic, particularly if you follow two simple principles. Firstly, keep calculations in the spreadsheet rather than in the macros – this keeps your working transparent to others. Secondly, use the record feature – by recording macros you can generate the code you need to perform different tasks without having to know how to write the code.

Macro commands are accessed from the *Tools > Macro* menu. Selecting 'Record new macro' from this menu starts the record feature. A pop-up box asks you to complete a name for the macro (no spaces allowed) after which a 'stop recording' button appears on your worksheet. From this point on, all actions that you perform will be converted to the equivalent visual basic code until you press the stop button. This is useful when you know what you want the macro to do, but not the code for how to do it, for example to record the costs and outcomes predicted by a probabilistic model each time the parameter values are simulated. These simulation results can then be stored for further analysis. In order to undertake the repetitive task of recording these results, we set up a simple loop.

To complement the record feature we need to know just two basic sets of commands. These are the 'Looping' commands and the ability to use relative cell referencing rather than absolute cell referencing.

In setting up a loop, we start by defining an index variable (Dim Index) and setting this index variable to zero (Index = 0) – this is our

Box 5.1: Example code for visual basic macro to record simulation results *(continued)*

counter variable. The basic loop starts with a 'Do' command and ends with a 'Loop' command. We then have a choice about how to incorporate the qualifying statement 'while' followed by a logical expression. Suppose that we want to undertake 1000 simulations. We can either specify 'Do While Index < 1000' in the first line of the loop, or we can specify 'Loop While Index <= 1000' in the last line of the loop. Remember to augment the counter variable in the penultimate line of the loop with a line of code: Index = Index + 1.

Suppose the purpose of the macro is to copy a probabilistic variable and record it to a results worksheet. If we record the copy and paste routine, the Visual Basic editor will default to using absolute cell referencing which specifies an alphanumeric code relating to the column (letter) and row (number) of the cell. If this is embedded within a loop then results will continually be pasted into the same cell. What we wish to do, however, is to record the results into different cells for each cycle of the loop. We therefore augment the code with a relative cell reference that specifies an offset of Y rows and X columns from a starting absolute cell reference. The code for this is shown below using the counter variable, Index, to offset an extra row for each cycle of the loop.

```
Range('G6').Select
ActiveCell.Offset(Index,0).Range('A1').Select
```

The first line sets the absolute reference and the second line specifies a relative reference using the absolute reference as a placeholder.

The code for this simple illustrative example is shown below as it would appear in the visual basic editor in Excel. Lines in bold indicate lines that were added (see above). The remaining lines can be recorded by carrying out the actions in Excel with the record feature on.

```
Sub Simulation()
Dim Index as Integer
Index = 0
    Do While Index < 1000
    Sheets('Results').Select
    Range('D10:E10').Select
    Selection.Copy
    Range('D18:E18').Select
```

Box 5.1: Example code for visual basic macro to record simulation results *(continued)*

```
    ActiveCell.Offset(Index,0).Range('A1').Select
    Selection.PasteSpecial Paste: = xlValues,
        Operation: = xlNone, SkipBlanks: = False,
        Transpose: = False
    Index = Index + 1
    Loop
End Sub
```

5.1.2. Interval estimates for cost-effectiveness ratios

With patient-level information on the costs and effects of treatment interventions it is natural to consider representing uncertainty in the ICER using interval estimates. Note that, as decision models are inherently Bayesian, it would be better to describe such intervals as 'credible intervals' rather then use the frequentist 'confidence interval'. We choose to talk about general 'interval' estimation, reflecting that the output parameters under discussion are from a decision model rather than statistical model.

Interval estimates can be obtained for outcomes of interest using the simulation results by using the percentile method. This simply involves taking the $\alpha/2$ and $(1 - \alpha/2)$ percentiles of the simulation vector as the $(1 - \alpha)100\%$ uncertainty interval for outcome of interest. Percentile intervals for the HIV/AIDS example are shown in Fig. 5.3, with the horizontal I-bar representing the 95 per cent uncertainty interval on life-years gained, the vertical I-bar representing the 95 per cent uncertainty interval on incremental cost, and the 'wedge' representing the 95 per cent uncertainty interval on the ICER.

5.1.3. Beyond interval estimation: acceptability curves

Although it was possible to calculate the 95 per cent uncertainty interval for the ICER in the case of the HIV/AIDS model as illustrated in Fig. 5.3, the overall level of uncertainty will often be such that problems are caused for interval estimation for the ICER. This occurs when simulation results cross the vertical axis suggesting that there is non-negligible probability that the new treatment is less effective than the existing treatment. The problem is that ratios of the same sign, but from different quadrants, are not strictly comparable. Negative ICERs in the NW quadrant of the plane (favouring the existing treatment) are

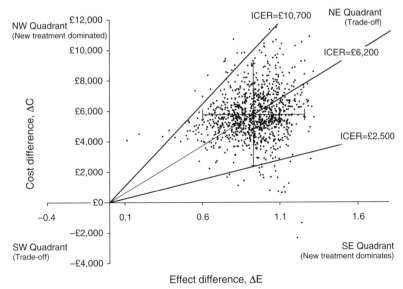

Fig. 5.3 Monte Carlo simulation results on the cost-effectiveness plane for the HIV/AIDS model showing interval estimates for cost, effect and incremental cost-effectiveness ratio.

qualitatively different from negative ICERs in the SE quadrant (favouring the new treatment) yet will be grouped together in any naïve rank-ordering exercise. Similarly, positive ratios of the same magnitude in the SW and NE quadrants have precisely the opposite interpretation from the point of view of the intervention under evaluation. This is because the decision rule in the SW quadrant is the opposite of that in the NE. For example, an ICER of 500 may be considered as supporting a new treatment in the NE quadrant if society has set a threshold ratio of 1000. In the SW quadrant, however, this value of the ICER would be considered as support of the existing treatment rather than the new treatment. Again, any naïve ranking exercise could easily conflate ICERs with the same magnitude but with different implications for decision making.

A solution to this problem can be found by returning to the original decision rule introduced in Fig. 5.1. If the estimated ICER lies below the threshold ratio λ, reflecting the maximum that decision makers are willing to invest to achieve a unit of effectiveness, then it should be implemented. Therefore, in terms of the Monte Carlo simulations on the cost-effectiveness plane in Fig. 5.3, we could summarize uncertainty by considering how many of the simulations fall below and to the right of a line with slope equal to λ, lending support to the cost-effectiveness of the intervention. Of course, the appropriate

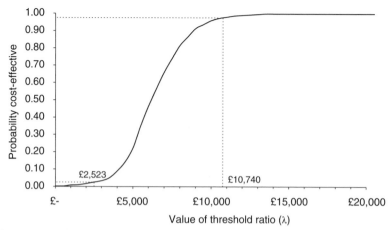

Fig. 5.4 Cost-effectiveness acceptability curve for the HIV/AIDS model showing the recovery of uncertainty interval estimates.

value of λ is itself unknown. However, it can be varied in order to show how the evidence in favour of cost-effectiveness of the intervention varies with λ. The resulting curve for the HIV/AIDS example is shown in Fig. 5.4 and has been termed a cost-effectiveness acceptability curve (van Hout *et al.* 1994) as it directly summarizes the evidence in support of the intervention being cost-effective (i.e. acceptable) for all potential values of the decision rule.

This 'acceptability curve' presents much more information on uncertainty than do confidence intervals. The curve cuts the horizontal axis at the probability that the intervention under evaluation is cost-saving, as a value of zero for λ implies that only the cost is important in the cost-effectiveness calculation. The curve is tending towards the probability that treatment is effective, as an infinite value for λ implies that effect only is important in the cost-effectiveness calculation. As well as summarizing, for every value of λ, the evidence in favour of the intervention being cost-effective, acceptability curves can also be employed to obtain the uncertainty interval on cost-effectiveness. The limits are obtained by looking across from the vertical axis to the curve at the appropriate points for the desired confidence level and reading off the associated cost-effectiveness value from the horizontal axis. For the HIV/AIDS example, we can recover the previously calculated interval of £2500/LYG to £10 700/LYG.

5.1.4. **The net-benefit framework**

Relatively recently, a number of researchers have employed a simple rearrangement of the cost-effectiveness decision rule in order to overcome the problems associated with ICERs (Claxton and Posnett 1996; Stinnett and Mullahy 1998; Tambour *et al.* 1998; Claxton 1999). In particular, Stinnett and Mullahy (1998) offer a comprehensive account of the net-benefit framework and make a convincing case for employing the net-benefit statistic to handle uncertainty in stochastic cost-effectiveness analysis. The algebraic formulation of the decision rule for cost-effectiveness analysis that a new treatment should be implemented only if its ICER lies below the threshold ratio, $\Delta C / \Delta E < \lambda$, can be rearranged in two equivalent ways to give two alternative inequalities on either the cost scale (net monetary benefit, NMB) (Claxton and Posnett 1996; Tambour *et al.* 1998; Claxton 1999) or on the effect scale (net health benefit, NHB) (Stinnett and Mullahy 1998):

$$NMB: \quad \lambda \cdot \Delta E - \Delta C > 0$$

$$NHB: \quad \Delta E - \frac{\Delta C}{\lambda} > 0.$$

These decision rules are entirely equivalent to the standard rule in terms of the ICER but have the advantage that when applying the net-benefit statistics to Monte Carlo simulation data, they will unambiguously sort out the 'acceptability' of an individual simulation trial on the cost-effectiveness plane. By using a net-benefit formulation, we can avoid the problem apparent with ICERs of conflating simulations of the same sign but in opposite quadrants of the cost-effectiveness plane. As such, it turns out to be much simpler to calculate acceptability curves from Monte Carlo simulations using net benefits than using the joint distribution of costs and effects.

The net-benefit framework also overcomes a particular problem associated with mean cost-effectiveness ratios. Introductory textbooks emphasize the importance of taking an incremental approach (Weinstein and Fineberg 1980; Drummond *et al.* 2005) rather than comparing mean cost-effectiveness ratios. A recent contribution to the literature highlighted the fundamental problem of taking patient-level mean ratios: the mean of ratios is not equal to the ratio of the mean values (Stinnett and Paltiel 1997). The consequence is that:

$$\frac{\bar{C}_1}{\bar{E}_1} - \frac{\bar{C}_0}{\bar{E}_0} \neq \frac{\bar{C}_1 - \bar{C}_0}{\bar{E}_1 - \bar{E}_0}$$

demonstrating that the incremental ratio cannot be constructed from the difference between the mean cost-effectiveness ratios in each arm of a trial or model.

By contrast, the difference in the average net-benefit of the experimental treatment and the average net-benefit of standard care treatment will give the overall incremental net-benefit statistic introduced above. This is straightforward to see algebraically through simple manipulation of the net-benefit expressions

$$N\bar{M}B_1 - N\bar{M}B_0 = \left(\lambda \cdot \bar{E}_1 - \bar{C}_1\right) - \left(\lambda \cdot \bar{E}_0 - \bar{C}_0\right)$$
$$= \lambda\left(\bar{E}_1 - \bar{E}_0\right) - \left(\bar{C}_1 - \bar{C}_0\right)$$
$$= \lambda \cdot \Delta\bar{E} - \Delta\bar{C}$$
$$= \Delta N\bar{M}B,$$

for the experimental (subscript 1) and control (subscript 0) interventions. Therefore the usefulness of the average net-benefit is not directly in terms of the average figures themselves, but in the simple linear relationship between average and incremental net-benefit. The full power of this simple relationship will become apparent subsequently when we turn to analysing multiple mutually exclusive treatment options.

5.2. Using ANCOVA to estimate the importance of individual parameters

The presentation of simulation results on the cost-effectiveness plane and the use of CEACs gives a useful impression of the overall uncertainty in a model. However, it may still be important to understand the relative effect of the different parameters in terms of contribution to this overall uncertainty.

In order to explore this issue, we need to record not only the 'output' parameters (the costs and effects of the different interventions), but also the input parameters that go into providing each simulation of the outputs. When we have both the inputs and outputs of the model recorded, there are three approaches that we might use to explore individual parameter uncertainty. We might summarize the correlations between the inputs and outputs. However, this is not a recommended approach as correlations can be high even if the overall variance induced is low. A better approach is to use analysis of covariance methods (ANCOVA) which can summarize the proportion of the variance in the output parameter 'explained' by variation in the input parameter. However, in its simple form, this assumes a linear relationship between inputs and outputs, such that for nonlinear models this approach is only an approximation.

Figure 5.5 shows an ANCOVA analysis for the HIV/AIDS model applied to both incremental cost only (left-hand side of figure) and incremental life-years gained only (right-hand side). Although the ANCOVA could also be applied to net-benefit conditional on a specific value of the threshold ratio, the results would reflect a middle ground between the two extremes shown

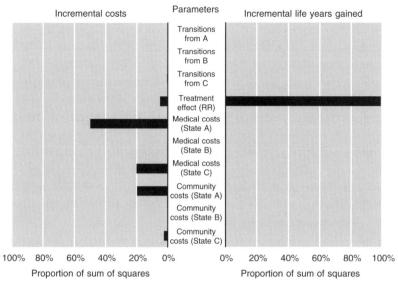

Fig. 5.5 ANCOVA analysis of proportion of sum of squares for incremental cost (left-hand side) and incremental life years gained (right-hand side) explained by uncertainty in the model input parameters.

in the figure. The figure clearly shows that the medical costs of states A and C, and the community care cost of state A in the model are most important for explaining the uncertainty of incremental cost. For incremental life years, only the treatment effect (expressed in the model as a relative risk) is important. Note that all of the transition probabilities from a given state of the model are grouped together, reflecting the fact that these are all estimated from a single Dirichlet distribution. For example, the 'transitions from A' include all four transition parameters from A to each of the other states in the model (including remaining in A) as these are all obtained from the same Dirichlet distribution. ANCOVA analysis easily allows grouping of related variables in this way. That the transition probabilities do not seem to impact the uncertainty in either incremental costs or effects reflects the relative precision with which these parameters of the model are estimated.

   Although the ANCOVA approach is only an approximation to the individual parameter contribution for nonlinear models, its ease of implementation has much to recommend it. Having recorded the input parameters and the corresponding output parameters of the model, it is a very simple step to run an ANCOVA for a given output parameter using the input parameters as explanatory variables. This can be done in any standard software package including many spreadsheet packages. Furthermore, the R^2 statistic provides a summary of the extent of approximation in nonlinear models (as for a linear model, the uncertainty in the inputs should perfectly explain the uncertainty in the outputs resulting in an R^2 of 100%).

It is important to recognize that an ANCOVA analysis only summarizes the individual parameter contribution to the variance of the output of interest (incremental costs, incremental effects or net-benefit) when our real concern is with decision uncertainty. In the next chapter, a more sophisticated approach based upon value-of-information methods will be introduced. This allows the individual parameter contribution to decision uncertainty to be assessed. Nevertheless, the straightforward nature of the ANCOVA approach is likely still to be useful for a swift understanding of the main parameter contributions to uncertainty in the model.

5.3. Representing uncertainty with multiple CEACs

In the AIDS/HIV example presented above, the presentation of the CEAC is perhaps the most common form found in the literature, with a single curve representing the incremental analysis of a new treatment alternative for an assumed homogeneous group of patients. However, it is often the case that patient characteristics can affect the potential outcomes of the model, such that treatment choices may be different for patients with different characteristics. Furthermore, it is rarely true that there is only one treatment alternative that is relevant for a single patient group. In this section, we provide an overview of the two distinct situations that may lead to the presentation of multiple acceptability curves in the same figure, representing rather different situations. These two situations reflect a common distinction in economic evaluation that governs how the incremental analysis is performed (Karlsson and Johannesson 1996; Briggs 2000). Where the same intervention can be provided to different patients, the decision to implement that intervention can be made independently based on the characteristics of the patient. This contrasts with the situation where different (though possibly related) interventions are possible treatment options for the same group of patients, such that a choice of one intervention excludes the others.

5.3.1. Multiple curves for patient subgroups (modelling heterogeneity)

In the past, many economic evaluations, including many cost-effectiveness modelling exercises, have assumed that patients eligible for treatment are essentially homogeneous. This approach has, most likely, been encouraged by the lack of memory in a Markov model, which fundamentally assumes that all patients in a given state are homogeneous, and due to the fact that most modelling exercises are based on secondary analyses with parameter estimates based on aggregated statistics across patient samples. In Chapter 4, much attention was given to the potential use of regression analysis to understand heterogeneity in parameter estimates. However, such analyses are dependent on the analyst having access to patient-level data.

Where patient characteristics influence the parameters of a model, then it is clear that the resulting cost-effectiveness can differ. Where the aim of cost-effectiveness analysis is to estimate the lifetime cost per quality-adjusted life-year (QALY) of an intervention, it should be clear that life expectancy will influence potential QALY gains and that this in turn is influenced by (among other things) the age and sex of the subject. Furthermore, health-related quality of life (HRQoL) is also dependent on age and possibly on sex, as is evident from the published HRQoL norms for the UK (Kind *et al.* 1999). Therefore, at the most fundamental level, we might expect heterogeneity in all cost-per-QALY figures even before considering heterogeneity in the parameters of the disease process, treatment effect and costs.

As it is possible to implement different treatment decisions for patients with different characteristics, all cost-effectiveness models should at least consider the potential for their results to vary across different subgroups and, in principle, each subgroup of patients should be represented by a different CEAC in order to facilitate different policy decisions. This general approach will be illustrated later in this chapter by showing how a series of statistical equations that model heterogeneity can be combined to estimate cost-effectiveness that varies by patient characteristics for a stable coronary disease population treated with an ACE inhibitor. Although the example relates to cardiovascular disease, the implications of heterogeneity are much more general and are likely to impact almost all potential evaluations. Indeed, true homogeneity of patient populations is rare and consideration should always be given as to whether different characteristics could result in different treatment decisions for different categories of patient.

5.3.2. Multiple curves for multiple treatment options

As argued above, the standard presentation of the CEAC reflects the standard concern of cost-effectiveness analysis with the incremental comparison of an experimental treatment against a comparator treatment. Similarly, in clinical evaluation, randomized control trials commonly have just two arms. However, it is rarely the case that decision makers face such a restricted set of options. Furthermore, in decision modelling (in direct contrast to clinical trial research) the cost of including additional options in an evaluation is small. As was argued in Chapter 1, economic evaluation should include all relevant treatment comparisons if they are to reliably inform decision making.

The consequence is that, in a fully specified economic model, there are likely to be more than two treatment alternatives being compared. When this is the case, multiple CEACs can be presented. These curves are conceptually the same as the use of acceptability curves to summarize uncertainty on the cost-effectiveness plane in a two-treatment decision problem except that there is now a curve relating to each treatment option.[1] The characterizing feature of the presentation of multiple CEACs to represent multiple and mutually exclusive treatment options is that the curves sum to a probability of one vertically.

Later in this chapter we will return to the example of gastro-oesophageal reflux disease (GORD) management introduced in Chapter 2 to illustrate the use of multiple CEACs in practice. Particular attention is given to the role of the mean net-benefit statistic as a tool for calculating the curves.

5.4. A model of the cost-effectiveness of ACE-inhibition in stable coronary heart disease (case study)

In this section, we describe a model for the treatment of stable coronary artery disease with an ACE-inhibitor. Of particular note is the use of regression methods (both parametric survival analysis and ordinary least squares) to represent heterogeneity following the methods outlined in Chapters 3 and 4. The model outlined has been described in detail elsewhere (technical report available from the authors) and the results have been published separately (Briggs *et al.* 2006). The model was constructed from data obtained from the EUropean trial on Reduction Of cardiac events with Perindopril in patients with stable coronary Artery disease (EUROPA) study. The trial randomized 12 218 patients with stable coronary heart disease to the ACE inhibitor perindopril 8 mg once daily or to matching placebo. Over a mean follow-up of 4.2 years, the trial showed that the use of perindopril resulted in a 20 per cent relative risk reduction in the primary endpoint of cardiovascular death, myocardial infarction or cardiac arrest (from a mean risk of 9.9 per cent in the placebo arm to 8.0 per cent in the perindopril arm) (The EUROPA Investigators, 2003).

---

[1] In the two alternative cases, the standard presentation of CEACs involves plotting the probability that the experimental observation under evaluation is cost-effective. Note, however, that the probability that the control intervention is cost-effective could be plotted, but would simply amount to the perfect complement of the first curve.

The model was designed to assess the cost-effectiveness of perindopril 8 mg once daily from the perspective of the UK National Health Service. Outcomes from treatment are assessed in terms of QALYs. The time horizon of the analysis was 50 years and costs and future QALYs were discounted at an annual rate of 3.5 per cent (NICE 2004). The majority of the data used in the analysis are taken from the EUROPA trial. An important objective of the analysis was to assess how cost-effectiveness varies according to patients' baseline risks of the primary EUROPA endpoints (nonfatal myocardial infarction, cardiac arrest or cardiovascular death – hereafter referred to as 'primary events').

5.4.1. Model structure

A Markov model was chosen as the preferred structure for the model and a state transition diagram for the Markov model of the EUROPA study is shown in Fig. 5.6. The general principle was to stay as close to the trial data as possible, therefore patients enter the model into the 'trial entry' state. Over the course of the model (employing a yearly cycle for 50 years until the vast majority of patients have died), patients are predicted to suffer a 'first event', which is represented by the rectangular box. This corresponds to the primary combined endpoint of the trial of cardiovascular mortality together with nonfatal myocardial infarction or cardiac arrest. Note that the use of the rectangular box is to emphasize that this is a predicted event and not a state of the model. Patients suffering events will either experience a fatal event, in which case they will move to the 'cardiovascular death' state, with the remainder deemed to have survived the event and so move to the 'nonfatal event history' state. In the

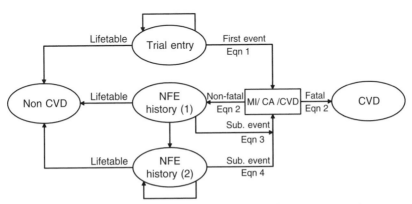

Fig. 5.6 State transition diagram for the Markov model of the EUROPA study. MI, myocardial infarction; CA, cardiac arrest; CVD, cardiovascular death; NFE, nonfatal event; non-CVD, noncardiovascular death.

first year after a nonfatal event, patients are assumed to have an elevated risk of a subsequent event. However, if patients do not experience a subsequent event, they move, in the next cycle (year) to a second 'nonfatal event history' state. From this state, they can again experience a subsequent event, but at a lower rate than the immediate year after the first event. From any of the states where patients are alive, they are deemed at a competing risk of a noncardio-vascular death.

With the addition of mean costs and HRQoL scores for each state as described above, the model was able to estimate expected (mean) costs and QALYs over a 50-year period for the perindopril and standard management options. The model assumes that perindopril is only potentially effective while it is being taken by patients. In the base case analysis it was assumed that patients would take the drug only for 5 years, after which they would not incur the costs of treatment. Once treatment stops, event rates are assumed to be the same for the two arms of the model.

5.4.2. Risk equations underlying the model

The analysis is based on a series of risk equations estimated using EUROPA data. These estimate the relationship between the primary event and patients' characteristics, including to which arm of the trial they were randomized. Of the 12 218 patients in the original EUROPA study, 292 did not have a complete set of data on covariates. The model development is therefore based on the 11 926 remaining patients for whom full information was available. With the addition of data from UK life tables on mortality rates for noncardiovascular reasons, the risk equations facilitate simulation of the fatal and nonfatal events that a cohort of patients is expected to experience with and without perindopril. The equations are based on a mean follow-up of 4.2 years in EUROPA, but the statistical relationships they represent are assumed to apply over the 50-year time horizon of the analysis. The mean costs and QALYs associated with the use of perindopril, relative to standard management, are estimated by attaching costs and HRQoL values to the events patients experience over time.

Three risk equations were estimated from the EUROPA data. The first is a standard parametric time-to-event survival analysis relating to the patient's risk of a first primary event following randomization. It is based on 1069 primary events observed in the 11 926 patients (592 in the placebo group and 477 in the perindopril group). The second equation is a logistic regression estimating the probability that a given first primary event would be fatal. This is based on the 1069 primary events of which 400 (38 per cent) were fatal. The third equation estimates the risk of a further primary event in the year following an initial nonfatal event, a period during which the data suggested a patient was at much higher risk of a subsequent event. The risk of a further primary event one or more years after the initial event is based on the first risk equation, updated to reflect the fact that all patients would have experienced a nonfatal event.

Table 5.1 presents the results of fitting each of these risk models, and shows which of a set of baseline risk factors were predictive in the equations (choice of predictive factors was based on a mix of statistical significance and clinical judgement). The first equation shows the hazard ratios associated with the risk of a first cardiac event (the trial primary endpoint of cardiovascular death, myocardial infarction or cardiac arrest). Of note is the 20 per cent risk reduction associated with being randomized to perindopril, as reported in the main trial report (The EUROPA investigators 2003).

Other characteristics found to be protective were younger age, being female, previous revascularization and cholesterol lowering therapy. Among characteristics found to increase risk were being a smoker, having had a previous myocardial infarction and symptomatic angina. The second equation shows a logistic regression estimating the odds of the first cardiac event being fatal. It can be seen that only three characteristics were important enough to enter this equation: being older, having had a previous myocardial infarction and increased levels of total cholesterol were all found to increase the odds of the event being fatal. Importantly, the use of perindopril was found not to influence the risk of the event being fatal. The third equation considered the risk of a subsequent event in the year after an initial event. Just one characteristic was found to be important in explaining this risk: the presence of angina symptoms (levels 2, 3 or 4 on the Canadian Cardiovascular Society's angina scale) or previous history of heart failure elevated the risk of a subsequent event. The ancillary parameter of the Weibull model was less than one, indicating a sharply falling hazard of subsequent events over time. The first equation is used to estimate the risk of subsequent primary events one or more years after an initial nonfatal event (with the nonfatal event covariate having been updated) as the trial itself had very little data in on the long-term risk of events subsequent to the first primary event. The assumption is that after the first year, patients will have stabilized and the risks of subsequent events will be similar to the risk of the first trial event. As this first equation also includes a treatment effect of perindopril, the model effectively assumes that continued treatment will reduce the risk of subsequent, as well as initial, events.

5.4.3. Quality-adjusted life-years

The mean difference in QALYs between perindopril versus placebo is the area between the two quality-adjusted survival curves; three elements are involved

Table 5.1 Estimated risk equations for the risk of a first primary event (equation 1), the odds of that event being fatal (equation 2) and the risk of a further primary event in the first year after a first nonfatal event (equation 3)

Explanatory baseline characteristics	Equation 1: Risk of first primary event (1069 events)*			Equation 2: Odds that first event is fatal (400 events)			Equation3 : Risk of subsequent event in first year following initial nonfatal event		
	Hazard ratio	Lower 95% limit	Upper 95% limit	Odds ratio	Lower 95% limit	Upper 95% limit	Hazard ratio	Lower 95% limit	Upper 95% limit
Use of perindopril	0.81	0.71	0.91						
Age in years				1.04	1.03	1.05			
Years greater than age 65	1.06	1.04	1.08						
Male	1.54	1.28	1.87						
Smoker	1.49	1.27	1.74						
Previous myocardial infarction	1.44	1.26	1.66	1.60	1.19	2.14			
Previous revascularization	0.88	0.77	0.99						
Existing vascular disease†	1.69	1.44	1.98						
Diabetes mellitus	1.49	1.28	1.74						
Family history of coronary artery disease	1.21	1.05	1.38						
Symptomatic angina‡ or history of heart failure	1.32	1.16	1.51				1.85	1.29	2.64

*Primary trial endpoint of cardiovascular mortality, myocardial infarction or cardiac arrest; †any of stroke, transient ischaemic attack or peripheral vascular disease

Table 5.1 (continued) Estimated risk equations for the risk of a first primary event (equation 1), the odds of that event being fatal (equation 2) and the risk of a further primary event in the first year after a first nonfatal event (equation 3)

Explanatory baseline characteristics	Equation 1: Risk of first primary event (1069 events)*			Equation 2: Odds that first event is fatal (400 events)			Equation 3: Risk of subsequent event in first year following initial nonfatal event		
	Hazard ratio	Lower 95% limit	Upper 95% limit	Odds ratio	Lower 95% limit	Upper 95% limit	Hazard ratio	Lower 95% limit	Upper 95% limit
Systolic blood pressure	1.00	1.00	1.01						
Units creatinine clearance below 80ml/min	1.01	1.00	1.02						
BMI > 30 (obese)	1.41	1.22	1.63						
Total cholesterol	1.13	1.07	1.20	1.21	1.08	1.35			
Using nitrates at baseline	1.42	1.25	1.63						
Using calcium channel blockers at baseline	1.20	1.06	1.36						
Using lipid lowering therapy at baseline	0.86	0.75	0.97						
Constant term (on the log scale)	−12.27	−12.97	−11.57	−4.37	−5.54	−3.20	−6.46	−7.25	−5.67
Ancillary parameter							0.70	0.59	0.82

*Primary trial endpoint of cardiovascular mortality, myocardial infarction or cardiac arrest; †any of stroke, transient ischaemic attack or peripheral vascular disease in this calculation. The first is the risk of cardiovascular mortality – this is based on the risk equations described above. The second is the mortality rate for noncardiovascular causes. This is based on official life tables for England and Wales and for Scotland (http://www.statistics.gov.uk/methods_quality/publications.asp), with deaths for cardiovascular reasons removed. Data are combined to give the rate of noncardiac death, by age and sex, for Great Britain. It is assumed that perindopril does not affect the mortality rate from noncardiovascular causes. Indeed, in the EUROPA trial, death from noncardiovascular causes was not significantly different (2.8% versus 2.6% for placebo and perindopril, respectively).

The third element in estimating QALYs is the HRQoL experienced by patients over time. Given that no HRQoL data were collected in EUROPA, the following approach was taken. Mean age- and sex-specific HRQoL scores for the UK population were identified based on the EQ-5D instrument, a generic instrument which provides an index which runs between 0 (equivalent to death) and 1 (equivalent to good health), where negative values are permitted, based on the preferences of a sample of the UK public (Kind *et al.* 1999). To represent the mean decrement in HRQoL associated with coronary heart disease, relative to the population mean, the mean baseline EQ-5D score measured in all patients in a trial comparing bypass surgery with coronary stenting was used (Serruys *et al.* 2001). Patients in this trial had a mean baseline age of 61 years and, on average, their HRQoL score was 14 per cent below the same aged group in the UK population. This decrement was employed to represent the HRQoL of all living patients in the analysis regardless of which cardiac events they had experienced.

5.4.4. Costs

Three elements of costs were included in the analysis, all of which are expressed in 2004 UK pounds. The first was the acquisition cost of perindopril. This was based on the use of 8 mg of perindopril once daily over a period of 5 years. Perindopril is costed at £10.95 per 30-tablet pack, or 37p per day, which represents its UK price from 1st January 2005 (Joint Formulary Committee 2005).

The second cost element related to concomitant medications, the use of which was recorded at each EUROPA follow-up visit, based on 13 cardiovascular categories. The British National Formulary (no.48) (Joint Formulary Committee 2004) was used to ascertain the typical individual drug preparations in each category and their recommended daily doses. The Department of Health's Prescription Cost Analysis 2003 database (Department of Health 2004) was used to estimate a mean daily cost for each of the concomitant drug categories.

The third element of costs related to days of inpatient hospitalization for any reason which were recorded at follow-up in EUROPA, together with ICD-9 codes on reasons for admission. In order to translate these data into costs, one of the clinical team, blinded to treatment allocation, mapped all relevant ICD-9 codes to UK hospital specialties. The cost per day for each specialty was taken from the UK Trust Financial Returns (NHS Executive 2004) which generated a cost for each hospitalization episode in EUROPA.

The implications of the cost of concomitant medications and inpatient hospitalizations for the cost-effectiveness of perindopril were assessed using a linear regression analysis. Its purpose was to estimate the mean costs associated with the events considered in the risk equations defined above – for example, to estimate the mean cost incurred in the year a patient experiences a first primary event. The covariates for the cost regression were selected using the same process as for the risk equations.

The regression analysis on costs is reported in Table 5.2 and indicates a 'background' annual cost per surviving patient that depends on age, presence of any existing disease, presence of angina symptoms, creatinine clearance and

Table 5.2 Results of the cost regression showing costs for the different model states and the impact of covariates

Explanatory variable	Cost (£)	Standard error	Lower 95% limit	Upper 95% limit
Nonfatal primary endpoint	9776	124	9533	10 019
History of nonfatal event	818	91	640	997
Fatal primary endpoint	3019	153	2719	3318
Non-CVD death	10 284	183	9924	10 643
Age	11	2	7	14
Existing vascular disease	326	47	234	418
Diabetes mellitus	215	43	131	298
Symptomatic angina	229	34	163	295
Units creatinine clearance below 80ml/min	7	2	3	10
Using nitrates at baseline	230	29	173	288
Using calcium channel blockers at baseline	152	30	93	211
Using lipid lowering therapy at baseline	95	28	40	150
Constant	−17	106	−225	192

the use of nitrates, calcium channel blockers or lipid lowering agents at baseline. In addition to these background costs, the regression model predicts the additional costs associated with the modelled events in the trial. In the year in which a nonfatal primary event occurs, £9776 is added to the background cost. In subsequent years, the addition to the background cost is £818. In the year that a fatal cardiovascular event occurs, the additional cost is estimated as £3019, which contrasts with an additional cost of £10 284 in the year of a noncardiovascular death. This difference can be explained by the fact that cardiovascular death is often relatively quick compared with other types of death. The advantage of this regression approach rather than just costing the events of interest is that the full cost to the health service is captured, including the 'background' costs of extending the life of patients.

5.4.5. Distributions for model parameters

Following the methods outlined in Chapter 4, the distributional assumptions are chosen to reflect the form of the data and the way in which the parameters were estimated. Standard statistical assumptions relating the estimation of the regression models were used for the risk equations. For the survival analysis models the assumption was multivariate normality of the log hazards scale. For the logistic regression model, the assumption was multivariate normality on the log odds scale. For the cost equation, the assumption was multivariate normality on the raw cost scale. In all cases, Cholesky decomposition of the variance–covariance matrices was used to capture correlation between coefficients in the regression models. For the population norms for EQ-5D, the assumption is normality within the age/sex-defined strata. For the assumption of 14 per cent reduction in utility, the assumption is a gamma distribution with variance equal to the mean reduction. No uncertainty is assigned for the risk of noncardiac death as these estimates are based on national death registers where the numbers are very large.

5.4.6. Representing parameter uncertainty and heterogeneity in the results of the EUROPA model

One of the main features of the modelling work described above is the direct modelling of heterogeneity between patients, in addition to the handling of uncertainty. These two aspects are presented separately below. Firstly, the results across different characteristics of patients in EUROPA are presented. Secondly, the importance of uncertainty for selected types of patient (based on their ranking of estimated cost-effectiveness) is illustrated.

Heterogeneity of cost-effectiveness within EUROPA

The cost-effectiveness model, structured as described above from a series of interlinking covariate adjusted risk equations and life tables, is able to predict cost-effectiveness as a function of the covariate pattern. Therefore, for each patient in EUROPA the cost-effectiveness model was used to generate a prediction of the cost-effectiveness for that set of patient characteristics based on a comparison of treating with perindopril versus not treating that type of patient. A histogram of the distribution of predicted cost-effectiveness results (in terms of incremental cost per QALY gained from perindopril) for each of the individuals in EUROPA is presented in Fig. 5.7. It is important to recognize that this distribution represents the estimated heterogeneity in the EUROPA study with regard to cost-effectiveness – it does not relate to uncertainty as the data points in Fig. 5.7 relate only to point estimates. This heterogeneity in cost-effectiveness arises from the heterogeneity of baseline risk of primary events combined with a constant relative risk reduction associated with treatment, resulting in differing absolute risk reductions for patients with different characteristics. The median (IQ range) cost-effectiveness across the heterogeneous population of EUROPA was estimated as £9500 per QALY (£6500–14 400) per QALY. Overall, 89 per cent of the EUROPA population were estimated to have a point estimate of incremental cost per QALY below £20 000 and 97 per cent below £30 000.

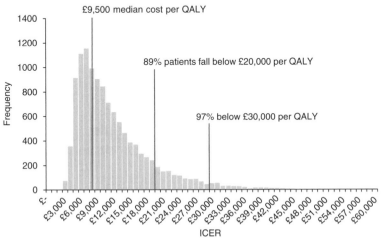

Fig. 5.7 Distribution of predicted cost-effectiveness results for individuals in the EUROPA study.

Probabilistic assessment of parameter uncertainty

As highlighted above, the analysis of heterogeneity was based only on point estimates of the cost-effectiveness of perindopril. As the model is based on a linked set of statistical equations, the probabilistic analysis is reasonably straightforward, being based on standard statistical assumptions concerning the distribution of parameters, as described previously. However, the need to separate out heterogeneity from uncertainty complicates the presentation. The approach taken is to illustrate uncertainty for five individuals, chosen on the basis of their location within a rank ordering of the cost-effectiveness results (the 2.5th, 25th, 50th (median), 75th and 97.5th percentiles). The 5-year risk of a primary trial endpoint and the covariate patterns for each of these individuals are set out in Table 5.3 along with the point estimates of incremental cost, QALYs gained and estimated cost per QALY ratio for these five individuals. These individuals are then used to illustrate uncertainty in the remainder of the section.

Propagating the statistical parameter uncertainty through the model for each of the individual covariate patterns presented in Table 5.3 generates an estimated joint distribution in the uncertainty of additional cost and QALY gain estimates. These are presented on the cost-effectiveness plane in Fig. 5.8 (for just the median, 2.5th and 97.5th percentiles from Table 5.3 for clarity). Each joint density plot is summarized by an acceptability curve (van Hout *et al.* 1994) in Fig. 5.9.

By effectively presenting uncertainty and heterogeneity on the same plot, these figures emphasize the importance of understanding the difference between the two concepts. In particular, note how the separate acceptability curve for each type of patient within Fig. 5.9 encourages the decision maker to make an independent treatment decision across different categories of patient, based on both the expected cost-effectiveness for that set of characteristics and the associated uncertainty.

5.5. Analysing simulation results: multiple treatment options

This section employs the model for assessing the cost-effectiveness of six management strategies for the treatment of GORD that was introduced in Chapter 2 in order to illustrate the issues that arise when evaluating multiple treatment options that are mutually exclusive for a given set of patients. Full details of the model have been presented in detail previously (Goeree *et al.* 1999; Briggs *et al.* 2002a), and so the focus of this section is on a discussion of the appropriate probabilistic assessment of the model.

Table 5.3 Illustrative cost-effectiveness results for five covariate patient profiles

	Percentile of ranked cost-effectiveness results				
	2.5th	25th	Median	75th	97.5th
Age in years	51	35	59	52	55
Male	1	1	1	1	1
Smoker	0	0	0	0	0
Previous myocardial infarction	1	1	0	1	0
Previous revascularization	1	0	1	1	1
Existing vascular disease	1	0	0	0	0
Diabetes mellitus	1	0	0	0	0
Family history of coronary artery disease	0	1	1	1	1
Symptomatic angina/history of heart failure	1	0	0	0	0
Systolic blood pressure	135	125	125	125	122
Creatinine clearance ml/min	74	125	109	108	76
BMI > 30 (obese)	0	0	0	1	0
Total cholesterol	4.2	6.3	6.6	3.7	4.48
Using nitrates at baseline	1	1	1	0	0
Using calcium channel blockers at baseline	0	0	1	0	0
Using lipid lowering therapy at baseline	0	1	0	1	1
Predicted 5-year risk of primary endpoint (%)	23	10	9	6	4
Incremental cost (£)	404	352	484	447	500
QALYs gained	0.108	0.054	0.051	0.031	0.016
Incremental cost-effectiveness ratio (£)	3700	6500	9500	14 400	32 100

5.5.1. A model for assessing the cost-effectiveness of GORD treatment

Gastro-oesophageal reflux disease is a common condition that results from regurgitation of acid from the stomach into the oesophagus. The most frequent symptom of GORD is heartburn and the majority of patients with GORD require pharmacotherapy to reduce acid secretion. Currently, the choice of first-line antisecretory therapy is between the H_2-receptor

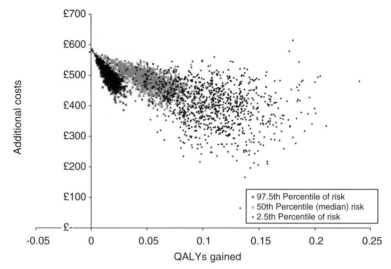

Fig. 5.8 Cost-effectiveness plane showing the scatter plot of 1000 Monte Carlo trials of the probabilistic model for the low, moderate and high-risk individuals from EUROPA.

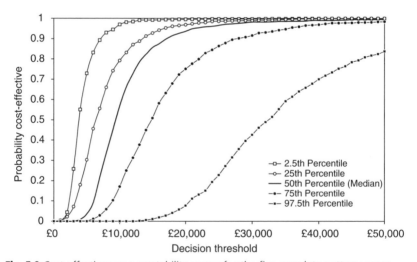

Fig. 5.9 Cost-effectiveness acceptability curves for the five covariate patterns representing percentile points from the cost-effectiveness distribution.

antagonists (H_2RAs), such as ranitidine and cimetidine, and proton pump inhibitors (PPIs) such as omeprazole. Although they have higher acquisition costs, PPIs have been found to be more efficacious than H_2RAs in terms of both the rate and speed of healing.

The objective of the original study was to compare, over a 1-year period, the expected costs and outcomes of alternative drug treatment strategies for the management of patients with erosive oesophagitis confirmed by endoscopy, but without complications such as Barrett's oesophagus or stricture. Outcomes are quantified in terms of GORD recurrence and weeks per year without GORD as indicated by data from clinical trials on healing and recurrence of oesophagitis.

Six strategies involving different combinations of first-line agents and change of therapy conditional on failure to heal or recurrence of GORD were modelled:

- Strategy A: Intermittent PPI. Acute treatment with a PPI for 8 weeks and then no further treatment with prescription medication until recurrence.

- Strategy B: Maintenance PPI. Acute treatment with a PPI for 8 weeks then continuous maintenance treatment with a PPI (same dose).

- Strategy C: Maintenance H_2RA. Acute treatment with an H_2RA for 8 weeks and then continuous maintenance treatment with an H_2RA (same dose).

- Strategy D: Step-down maintenance prokinetic agent. Acute treatment with a prokinetic agent (PA) for 12 weeks and then continuous maintenance treatment with a lower dose of PA.

- Strategy E: Step-down maintenance H_2RA. Acute treatment with a PPI for 8 weeks and then continuous maintenance treatment with a H_2RA.

- Strategy F: Step-down maintenance PPI. Acute treatment with a PPI for 8 weeks and then continuous maintenance treatment with a lower dose PPI.

Treatment options A–F represent clinical strategies rather than single drug treatments for the management of erosive oesophagitis where the physician is assumed to increase the dose of a drug or switch to another drug if the patient fails to respond to the first-line treatment. The structure of the decision tree that was developed was shown in Fig. 2.1. The model is recursive in two 6-month periods; hence, probabilities of recurrence in the period to 12 months are conditional upon recurrence or nonrecurrence in the period from 0 to 6 months.

Treatment outcomes

For GORD, the most commonly used formulation of outcome for economic evaluation has been either oesophagitis-free or symptom-free time in a period of follow-up. The advantage of such a measure is that it combines two important aspects of efficacy: (i) the speed with which oesophagitis is healed; and (ii) the likelihood of oesophagitis recurring. In this analysis, the primary outcome measure is GORD-free time during the 12-month period of the model, defined as the time where the oesophagitis is healed. A meta-analysis of healing and recurrence studies published to November 1997 was undertaken to estimate healing and recurrence probabilities together with associated GORD-free time. Full details of this analysis are given in the original study (Goeree *et al.* 1999).

Resource use and unit costs

Generic prices were used for drugs where a generic equivalent is available, employing the 'best available price' from the Ontario Drug Benefit (ODB) programme together with a 10 per cent pharmacy mark-up charge. A dispensing fee of Can$4.11 was used (i.e. ODB programme fee of Can$6.11 less a Can$2.00 patient co-payment). Cost estimates for physician fees were taken from the physician fee schedule for Ontario, and procedure costs, such as endoscopy, were estimated from a hospital participating in the Ontario Case Costing Project in Southwestern Ontario.

To estimate the costs associated with the management of patients with symptoms of GORD recurrence, information on clinical practice patterns and resource utilization was obtained by convening an expert physician panel and using a modified Delphi technique. Estimated resource utilization was then combined with unit cost information to give the mean cost associated with each recurrence under each management strategy.

5.5.2. Results from the GORD model

Before demonstrating the probabilistic assessment of multiple treatment options, the standard approach to generating a cost-effectiveness frontier of mutually exclusive options is reviewed.

Deterministic cost-effectiveness acceptability

The decision tree model outlined in Fig. 2.1 was evaluated to estimate the expected costs and the expected weeks without GORD in the 12-month period of the model. The conventional approach to examining the cost-effectiveness of the alternative strategies involves first determining whether any strategies are strictly dominated by other strategies having both lower costs and greater therapeutic effects, and secondly determining whether any strategies were dominated through the principles of extended dominance, that is, whether linear combinations of other strategies can produce greater benefit at lower cost (Cantor 1994). Then, among nondominated treatment options, incremental cost-effectiveness ratios are calculated by comparing each option with the next more costly and more effective intervention. This process produces an 'efficiency frontier' of increasingly more costly and more effective strategies. The results of this analysis for the GORD model are presented on the cost-effectiveness plane in Fig. 2.2, which also shows the efficiency frontier between nondominated options.

The figure clearly shows that step-down maintenance PA (strategy D) is dominated by maintenance H_2RA, (strategy C), intermittent PPI (strategy A) and step-down maintenance H_2RA (strategy E). The efficiency frontier is given by the lines joining strategies C (the origin) A, E and B. Strategy F is internal to this frontier indicating that it also can be ruled out through the principle of extended dominance (i.e. a linear combination of strategies E and B would strongly dominate F). The slope of the frontier at any point reflects incremental cost-effectiveness – the additional cost at which additional effects can be purchased.

Probabilistic assessment of the GORD model

Following the principles outlined in Chapter 4, distributions were specified for all the relevant parameters of the model – the details of which can be found in the original article (Briggs *et al.* 2002*b*). The probabilistic analysis was undertaken by randomly sampling from each of the parameter distributions and calculating the expected costs and expected weeks free from GORD for that combination of parameter values. This process formed a single replication of the model results and a total of 10 000 replications were performed in order to examine the distribution of the resulting cost and outcomes for each strategy. The results of these 10 000 replications from the model are presented on the cost-effectiveness plane in Fig. 5.10 together with the baseline estimate of the efficient frontier.

For each of the individual replications, an efficient frontier could be calculated together with the incremental cost-effectiveness ratios for treatments on the frontier. In particular, Fig. 5.10 suggests that it may not be possible to rule out strategy F, the strategy based on step-down maintenance PPI, as it potentially forms part of the frontier in many replications. Note, however, that it is impossible to gain a clear view from Fig. 5.10 as to how often strategy F forms part of the frontier. This is because there can be substantial covariance between the simulations plotted in the figure (it turns out that strategy F forms part of the frontier in 27 per cent of simulations although it is not clear how this result should be interpreted). The potential for covariance between simulation points limits the usefulness of presenting simulation results for multiple strategies on the cost-effectiveness plane. Only for cases such as

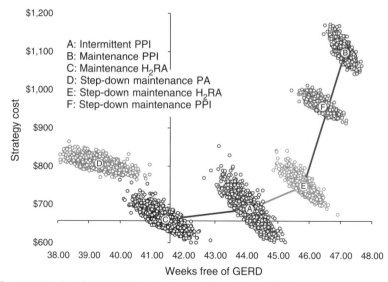

Fig. 5.10 Results of 10 000 Monte Carlo simulation evaluations of the gastro-oesophageal reflux disease model presented on the cost-effectiveness plane.

strategy D where there is clear separation of the (marginal) probability densities is it possible to draw a firm conclusion. Note, for example, that it would be impossible to infer the slope of any points along the simulated cost-effectiveness frontiers as it is not clear which simulated points should be joined together. For this reason we would suggest that the cost-effectiveness plane is not the appropriate vehicle for presenting simulation output for more than two treatment options.

Of course, it is possible to analyse the simulation results appropriately as this covariance information is recorded. Conditional on knowing the threshold ratio – in this example the willingness to pay for a week free from GORD symptoms – it is possible to identify the efficient frontier, calculate the incremental cost-effectiveness ratios and choose one strategy from the six available for each of the 10 000 replications. However, the application of the traditional construction of a cost-effectiveness frontier is rather involved and it turns out that a more straightforward approach exists, which is simple to implement for large numbers of simulation results.

This illustration of the usual case for two treatment alternatives is easily generalized to the multiple option case: the management option of choice from the six strategies under evaluation in the GORD example will be the option with the greatest mean net-benefit. This must be the case, as only that treatment will have a positive incremental net-benefit when compared with any other treatment alternative. The proportion of times a strategy has the highest net-benefit among the 10 000 replications of the model gives the strength of evidence in favour of that strategy being cost-effective. This ability of the net-benefit framework to handle multiple mutually exclusive treatment options is a very strong advantage of the approach and provides a much more straightforward solution to finding the cost-effective option from among multiple treatment alternatives than the conventional approach outlined above. We simply formulate the mean net-benefit for each option and choose the option with the greatest mean net-benefit. Only this option will have a positive incremental net-benefit relative to any other option. Note that there is no need to consider dominance (strict or extended) and there is no need to specify the appropriate comparator. Therefore it is very easy to implement in a form that can automatically find the optimal option in a large simulation experiment.

For example, ten simulations from the GORD model of six management options are shown in Table 5.4. The corresponding net-benefit for each option is shown on the left-hand side of Table 5.5, assuming a willingness to pay of $200 per week free from GORD symptoms. The indicator for whether a strategy is optimal is shown on the right-hand side of the table and corresponds to an indicator of whether the option has the highest mean net-benefit among all the options.

In reality, of course, the threshold ratio for a week free from GORD symptoms is not known. However, by plotting out the proportion of times the intervention has the greatest net-benefit, for all possible values of λ, much can be learned concerning the implications of the estimated uncertainty for the treatment decision. This generates a series of CEACs for the multiple option case. To calculate these CEACs, we have only to average across the trials to find the proportion of times that each option is optimal for a given ceiling ratio. We then repeat the process with a new threshold ratio and plot the results.

Figure 5.11 shows the result of just such an exercise for the probabilistic evaluation of the GORD model. Note the use of the log scale for the threshold ratio to help present the curves more clearly and also note that the summation across the curves at any point gives a total of one: this must be the case as the options are mutually exclusive.

As expected, strategy D does not feature in Fig. 5.11, indicating that it is never a contender for cost-effectiveness. Strategy F does feature, although it never achieves more than 13 per cent of simulations, suggesting it is cost-effective, even at the most favourable threshold ratio (about $260 per day free from GORD symptoms).

Table 5.4 Example of ten simulations of the six different management options

A		B		C		D		E		F	
SFWks	Cost ($)	SFWks	Cost ($)	SFWks	Cost ($)	SFWks	Cost ($)	SFWks	Cost ($)	SFWks	Cost ($)
43.96	714	47.00	1116	41.78	649	38.95	825	46.05	738	46.49	959
44.34	642	47.18	1085	40.92	671	39.63	799	45.50	753	46.60	936
44.37	695	47.22	1100	42.33	634	39.54	822	46.29	727	46.29	982
44.17	667	47.10	1097	40.82	679	39.02	816	45.47	762	46.43	949
44.01	676	47.12	1091	42.17	622	39.03	799	45.94	726	46.40	948
44.14	709	47.42	1079	41.10	693	39.62	813	45.69	773	46.56	961
44.21	692	47.26	1109	41.69	656	39.42	807	46.06	740	46.72	950
44.41	719	46.99	1130	41.59	681	39.09	840	46.06	766	46.51	978
44.27	693	47.18	1088	40.69	717	40.72	804	45.36	796	46.68	950
44.59	651	47.46	1083	40.66	717	39.39	809	45.35	792	46.66	953

SFWks, symptom free weeks

Table 5.5 Net benefits of each strategy and indicator showing whether strategy is optimal for the ten simulation of Table 5.4

Net benefits of each strategy ($)						Optimal?					
A	B	C	D	E	F	A	B	C	D	E	F
8078	8284	7708	6965	8472	8340	0	0	0	0	1	0
8226	8350	7513	7127	8348	8383	0	0	0	0	0	1
8179	8344	7832	7087	8532	8275	0	0	0	0	1	0
8166	8323	7485	6987	8331	8338	0	0	0	0	0	1
8125	8333	7811	7007	8462	8332	0	0	0	0	1	0
8119	8406	7526	7111	8365	8350	0	1	0	0	0	0
8151	8344	7683	7077	8472	8395	0	0	0	0	1	0
8163	8269	7638	6978	8446	8324	0	0	0	0	1	0
8161	8348	7421	7340	8277	8386	0	0	0	0	0	1
8268	8408	7415	7070	8277	8379	0	1	0	0	0	0

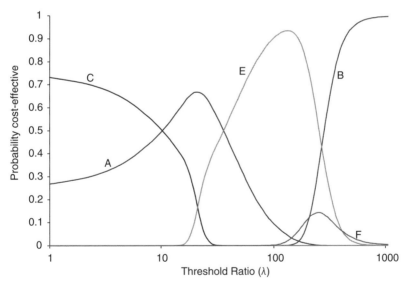

Fig. 5.11 Acceptability curves for the choice of treatment strategy (a log scale is employed to better illustrate the low values).

While this sort of presentation of the choice between mutually exclusive treatments in the face of many options is a natural extension of the use of CEACs in the two treatment cases, the issue arises of how exactly decision makers should use this information to choose between the remaining strategies that form part of the frontier. One approach would be to say that, for any given value of the shadow price, the optimal decision would be to choose the strategy that is most likely to be cost-effective. But of course, this decision rule gives the exact same treatment recommendations as the baseline estimates in Fig. 2.2, where uncertainty was not considered. Furthermore, Fenwick and colleagues (2001) have pointed out that such an approach is not consistent with maximizing net-benefit, if the distribution of net-benefit is skewed. Instead, they propose presenting the 'cost-effectiveness acceptability frontier', which is plotted for the GORD example in Fig. 5.12. The frontier shows the options that would be chosen under the rule of maximizing net-benefit, and although it closely accords with an approach of choosing the option that has the maximum probability of being cost-effective, there are some discrepancies.

For example, if the willingness to pay to avoid GORD symptoms was $270, then due to the skew in the distribution of net-benefit, strategy B is preferred to strategy E in terms of expected net-benefit, despite the fact that strategy E has a higher probability of being cost-effective.

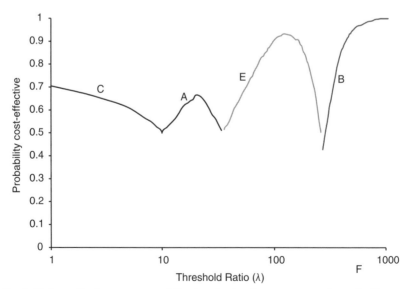

Fig. 5.12 Cost-effectiveness acceptability frontier for the gastro-oesophageal reflux disease example.

It is important to note that in moving towards the use of acceptability curves to represent uncertainty in treatment decisions, we are encouraging analysts and decision makers to think beyond conventional error rates in standard statistical analysis to guide decision making. It is clear from the curves in Fig. 5.11 that no options can be distinguished at the 95 per cent level of uncertainty within a reasonable range of willingness to pay for a week free from GORD. Of course, the arbitrary nature of the conventional approach to decision making under uncertainty emphasizes the inadequacies of such a simple decision rule based on statistical significance, indeed, Claxton (1999) has argued that significance testing of this sort is irrelevant. Instead he suggests that decision making should be fundamentally concerned with expected values. That is not to say that the decisions should be made on the basis of the baseline point estimates as presented in Fig. 2.2 without reference to uncertainty in obtaining those estimates. Rather, that the expected returns to obtaining further information should be assessed in order to determine whether it is worth commissioning more research to obtain improved estimates of the decision parameters and it is to this issue that we turn in the next chapter.

5.6. **Summary**

In summary, probabilistic modelling of deterministic models is a practical solution to the problems of conventional simple sensitivity analysis. Presenting uncertainty as CEACs encourages analysts and users to think carefully about the state of evidence relating to the parameters of the model. The use of acceptability curves to present information on the probability of multiple treatment options being cost-effective is a natural extension of the 'two alternatives' case usually presented in the literature. We will argue in the next chapter that an appropriate approach to decision making under uncertainty requires an understanding of the value of collecting additional information to inform decision making and that CEACs are not sufficient tools on their own. Nevertheless, it should become clear in the next chapter that expected value of information methods will have to be predicated on a well specified probabilistic model.

5.7. **Exercise: Analysing simulation results from the total hip replacement model**

5.7.1. **Overview**

The purpose of this exercise is to show how Excel can be used to run simulations drawing from the distributions chosen for the previously constructed probabilistic model of total hip replacement (Exercise 4.8) using macros to record the results.

The step-by-step guide covers four main areas:

1. Structuring the simulation and writing macros.

2. Analysing results: the cost-effectiveness plane.

3. Another macro for calculating CEACs.

4. Multiple curves: different patient subgroups.

The template for this exercise is '*Exercise 5.7 – template.xls*'.

5.7.2. **Step-by-step guide**

1. Structuring the simulation and writing macros

In the template file you will find a new worksheet *<Simulation>*. This sheet provides the structure for much of this exercise. The aim is to record repeated results from the probabilistic analysis constructed in Exercise 4.8 and to analyse the results. Results of each round of simulations (trials) are to be placed in rows, while columns record results for each trial.

    i. Note that columns C to O are labelled with parameter names. The aim here is to record the input parameter values along with the overall cost-effectiveness results (in columns Q to T). The first task is to link the cell under the parameter label with the relevant probabilistic parameter (first making sure that the 'probabilistic switch' is set to 1). Although you could do this by pointing to the live cells of the *<Parameters>* sheet, the most straightforward method is to use the parameter names.

    ii. Now do the same with the cost and effect output parameters.

By this stage, the row 4 for columns C to T should contain the corresponding probabilistic parameter. These cells should update to new parameters when the <F9> key is pressed – providing the 'switch cell' on the *<Parameters>* worksheet (D3) is set to 1. The next step is to construct a macro that will copy row 4 and paste it into the rows below 1000 times from row 6 to row 1005. You may find it useful to refer to Box 5.1 relating to macro writing.

    iii. Start by setting a new macro to record from the *Tools > Macro* menu.

    iv. First enter 1 in the 'switch' cell D3 on the *<Parameters>* worksheet to make sure the model is in probabilistic mode.
Hint: do this even if it is already set at 1, as the purpose is to record the action.

    v. Now switch to the *<Simulation>* worksheet and select cells C4:T4 and copy and paste these cells to row 6. Remember to use the *paste special* command in order to paste only the values and not the formulae.

    vi. Finally, set the switch cell back to 0 so that the model is in deterministic mode.

vii. Now use the on-screen button to stop the macro (this should have opened in a separate window when you started recording – if it did not for any reason, you need to stop the macro using the *Tools > Macro > Stop Recording* menu).

viii. Open the Visual Basic Editor (from the *Tools > Macro* menu) and you will find that the basics of your macro have been recorded for you. As demonstrated in Box 5.1, you need to add a variable to count the number of trials (1000), a Do Loop and an Active Cell Offset.

When complete, set your macro running from the *Tools > Macro > Run Macro* menu and your macro should repeatedly copy row 4 into the 1000 rows below – this is the result of the probabilistic sensitivity analysis that can now be analysed.

Note, you may want to examine the code in the solution file to see how to turn off the screen updating so that the macro runs in the background without showing the actions and causing the annoying 'screen flicker' effect.

2. Analysing the results: the cost-effectiveness plane

Now that we have the results of 1000 probabilistic trials of the model, the results can be analysed.

i. Begin by calculating the incremental cost and effect results (columns U and V of the *<Simulation>* worksheet) for each trial from the cost and effect in each arm of the model.

ii. Now plot these incremental results on the cost-effectiveness plane. Either plot them directly, or use the *<CE plane>* worksheet, where some of the formatting has been done for you.

Notice the slightly strange shape of the 'cloud' of points. This is due to the nonlinearity relating input and output parameters inherent in the model structure. As a consequence, the point estimates from the deterministic model (evaluated at the mean values of the distributions) are not the same as the expectations across the output parameters.

iii. In cells Q1007:V1007 calculate the mean values across the 1000 trials of the model.

iv. Now link the probabilistic results table on the *<Analysis>* sheet to these results and compare with the deterministic results (ensuring that the model is in deterministic mode).

You should notice that the probabilistic results are slightly different from the deterministic results. In fact, as argued in Chapter 4, it is the expectation across the probabilistic results that should be used as point estimates.

3. Another macro for calculating CEACs

Once probabilistic results are obtained as in the form of the first step above, the analysis of the results can proceed much like the analysis of bootstrap replications of real data in a statistical analysis (Briggs and Fenn 1998). This includes the potential for calculating confidence intervals for the ICER (using, for example, simple percentile methods) or CEACs. We focus on the calculation of CEACs as the appropriate way of presenting uncertainty in cost-effectiveness acceptability as a method that avoids the problems that can arise when uncertainty covers all four quadrants of the cost-effectiveness plane.

The calculation of CEACs will involve another macro (not essential, but useful in this context).[2] However, some preparation of the worksheet is required first. In particular, the presentation mentioned that two alternative approaches to the use of the net-benefit statistic could be used to generate acceptability curves. This exercise will calculate both in order to demonstrate that the methods are equivalent.

    i. On worksheet *<Simulation>* cell Z1 contains the 'threshold ratio' (i.e. the maximum acceptable willingness to pay for health gain). Use this value to calculate the mean net monetary benefit in columns X and Y for the standard and new prostheses, respectively (that is, using the costs and effects for the standard prosthesis from columns Q and R, and similarly for the new prosthesis).

    ii. In column Z, calculate in the incremental net monetary benefit of the new prosthesis using the incremental costs and effects from columns U and V.

    iii. In columns AB and AC use an IF(…) function to generate an indicator variable to show a value of 1 if the prosthesis (standard and new, respectively) is the most cost-effective for that trial, 0 if it is not. Remember, the most cost-effective prosthesis has the greatest *average* net-benefit.

    iv. In column AD use an IF(…) function to generate an indicator variable to show whether the new prosthesis is cost-effective compared with the standard prosthesis. This occurs when the *incremental* net-benefit of the new treatment is positive.

    v. Finally, calculate the mean of columns AB, AC and AD in row 4. This represents the proportions of simulation trials in which the associated prosthesis is cost-effective given the value of the ceiling ratio in cell Z1.

---

[2] For example, it is possible to create CEACs in Excel by using the 'data table' command. The disadvantage of this method, however, is that it includes large amounts of 'active' cells to the spreadsheet, all of which recalculate whenever an action is undertaken. In large models this can greatly increase the time it takes to run simulations,

Notice that columns AB and AC are direct complements of one another. As in the simple two treatment alternatives case, if one treatment is not cost-effective, then the other must be. Also notice that columns AC and AD give the same results for the new prosthesis. This is because the difference between average net benefits is the incremental net-benefit.

As the results in AB4:AD4 have been linked to the threshold ratio cell Z1, a simple macro can be used to change the value in Z1 and to record the corresponding results.

    vi. Start by selecting a new macro to record from the *Tools > Macro* menu.

    vii. First copy the value of the ceiling ratio from cell AF6 to Z1.

    viii. Now copy the results from AB4:AD4 to AG6:AI6 remembering to specify *paste special: values*.

    ix. Now stop the macro using the on-screen button and open the Visual Basic Editor.

    x. The basics of your macro have been recorded for you – in the same way as before you need to add a variable to count the number of ceiling ratio iterations (58), a Do Loop and an Active Cell Offset.

    xi. Once the macro has worked its magic, you can plot the resulting CEAC using the *<CEA Curve>* worksheet. Plot both the standard and new prosthesis curves.

4. Multiple curves: different patient subgroups

Up to this point we have been working with a model where the patient characteristics have been set for a female aged 60 years. In this part of the exercise, we want you to repeatedly obtain results for men and women aged 40, 60 and 80 years and record the results and present them as multiple acceptability curves.

    i. Your worksheet should already have the results for women aged 60. Copy and paste both the (probabilistic) point estimates and the CEAC results (for the new prosthesis only) into the table template in the appropriate point in the *<Sub-group results>* worksheet.

    ii. Now change the patient characteristics on the *<Analysis>* worksheet and re-run both your simulation and CEAC macros.
    Hint: you could set up a button to do this automatically and even link the two macros together with a single macro. Also make sure that you provided a sheet reference to your CEAC macro – otherwise running it from another sheet can have devastating results!

    iii. Finally, plot the resulting CEACs for the different patient characteristics on the *<Sub-group CEACs>* worksheet.

You should find that the curves can be quite different for different patient characteristics. For example, the new prosthesis seems to be more cost-effective generally for men (due to the fact that on average men have higher failure rates and so the absolute benefits of reducing failure risk are greater) and that the new prosthesis is not so cost-effective for elderly patients (where death is an important competing risk for prosthesis failure).

5.8. Exercise: introducing a third prosthesis into the total hip replacement model

5.8.1. Overview

The purpose of this exercise is to introduce a further prosthesis into the THR model in order to illustrate the approach to calculating multiple CEACs for multiple treatment options.

The step-by-step guide covers two main tasks:

1. Adding in a third prosthesis option.

2. Multiple curves for mutually exclusive treatment options.

The template for this exercise is '*Exercise 5.8 – template.xls*'.

5.8.2. Step-by-step guide

1. Adding in a third prosthesis option

Although in the vast majority of trials just two treatment alternatives are compared, in modelling it is much more common to look at multiple treatment options. If you open *Exercise 5.8 – template.xls*, you will find that an additional worksheet *<NP2>* has been added that contains the model for a second new prosthesis. Take a moment to examine the *<Hazard function>* worksheet, which contains additional information concerning this prosthesis in terms of its effectiveness and correlation with other parameters.

The aim in this section is to update the model so that the third prosthesis option is fully integrated. This involves updating the parameter, analysis and simulation sheets before re-running the probabilistic sensitivity analysis.

   i. Starting with the *<Hazard function>* worksheet, update the last row of the Cholesky decomposition matrix (row 32). Also update the last row of the random variable generating table (row 41).

   ii. Move to the *<Parameters>* worksheet and add in the information concerning the effectiveness of the new prosthesis in row 28.

iii. On the *<Simulation>* worksheet, link the input and output parameters in F4 and U4:V4 to the relevant cells (note that the naming has already been done for you).

iv. The simulation macro has already been edited to take into account the wider range of results to be recorded (C4:V4) so you can now run the 'MCsimulation' macro.

Now that the adaptations relating to the third option are complete the updated results can be produced.

v. Calculate the mean values across the simulations in cells Q1007:V1007 of the *<Simulation>* worksheet and use these values to update the point estimates for the probabilistic analysis on the *<Analysis>* worksheet.

vi. Plot the three options on the cost-effectiveness plane using the *<CE plane>* worksheet. (Note that you should do this by plotting three point clouds from columns Q to V, rather than plotting increments).

Note that one of the problems of looking at the three clouds of points on the cost-effectiveness plane is that we lose the perception of how the points are correlated between the three options.

2. Multiple curves for mutually exclusive treatment options

The results from the probabilistic analysis of mutually exclusive options can be presented as multiple acceptability curves. However, in contrast to the independent subgroup analysis of the first part of this exercise, these multiple curves must sum to one. We must therefore repeat the analysis based on net-benefit, but this time for three options, which is where the use of mean net-benefit becomes useful.

i. Calculate the average net monetary benefit for each option in columns X to Z.

ii. Now create indicator variables in columns AB to AD to show whether each of the three prostheses are cost-effective for that trial (only the prosthesis with the greatest net-benefit is cost-effective).

iii. Calculate the proportions of trials in which each of the prostheses are cost-effective in AB4:AD4.

iv. Now run the 'CEACurve' macro, which will generate the data for the acceptability curves in columns AF to AI.

v. Finally, plot the three acceptability curves using the worksheet *<CEA curve>*.

As was noted previously, the interpretation of multiple acceptability curves can be tricky – especially when the model is nonlinear. Fenwick *et al.* (2001)

have argued for the use of a cost-effectiveness acceptability frontier in these situations. An example of this applied to the model you have just constructed can be downloaded from the book website.

References

Black, W. C. (1990) 'The CE plane: a graphic representation of cost-effectiveness', *Medical Decision Making*, 10: 212–214.

Briggs, A. H. (2000) 'Handling uncertainty in cost-effectiveness models', *PharmacoEconomics*, 17: 479–500.

Briggs, A. and Fenn, P. (1998) 'Confidence intervals or surfaces? Uncertainty on the cost-effectiveness plane', *Health Economics*, 7: 723–740.

Briggs, A. H., Goeree, R., Blackhouse, G. and O'Brien, B. J. (2002*a*) 'Probabilistic analysis of cost-effectiveness models: choosing between treatment strategies for gastroesophageal reflux disease', *Medical Decision Making*, 22: 290–308.

Briggs, A. H., Goeree, R., Blackhouse, G. and O'Brien, B. J. (2002*b*) 'Probabilistic analysis of cost-effectiveness models: choosing between treatment strategies for gastroesophageal reflux disease', *Medical Decision Making*, 22: 290–308.

Briggs, A. H., Mihaylova, B., Sculpher, M., Hall, A., Wolstenholme, J., Simoons, M., Ferrari, R., Remme, W. J., Bertrand, M. and Fox, K. (2006) 'The cost-effectiveness of perindopril in reducing cardiovascular events in patients with stable coronary artery disease using data from the EUROPA Study', *Heart* 92(Suppl 2):A36.

Cantor, S. B. (1994) 'Cost-effectiveness analysis, extended dominance and ethics: a quantitative assessment', *Medical Decision Making*, 14: 259–265.

Chancellor, J. V., Hill, A. M., Sabin, C. A., Simpson, K. N. and Youle, M. (1997) 'Modelling the cost effectiveness of lamivudine/zidovudine combination therapy in HIV infection', *PharmacoEconomics*, 12: 54–66.

Claxton, K. (1999) 'The irrelevance of inference: a decision-making approach to the stochastic evaluation of health care technologies', *Journal of Health Economics*, 18: 341–364.

Claxton, K. and Posnett, J. (1996) 'An economic approach to clinical trial design and research priority-setting', *Health Economics*, 5: 513–524.

Department of Health (2004) *Prescription cost analysis: England 2003*, London, Department of Health.

Drummond, M. F., Sculpher, M. J., O'Brien, B., Stoddart, G. L. and Torrance, G. W. (2005) *Methods for the economic evaluation of health care programmes*, 3rd edn. Oxford, Oxford University Press.

Fenwick, E., Claxton, K. and Sculpher, M. (2001) 'Representing uncertainty: the role of cost-effectiveness acceptability curves', *Health Economics*, 10: 779–787.

Goeree, R., O'Brien, B., Hunt, R., Blackhouse, G., Willan, A. and Watson, J. (1999) 'Economic evaluation of long-term management strategies for erosive oesophagitis', *PharmacoEconomics*, 16: 679–697.

Joint Formulary Committee (2004) *British national formulary 48*. London, British Medical Association and Royal Pharmaceutical Society of Great Britain.

Joint Formulary Committee (2005) *British national formulary 49*. London, British Medical Association and Royal Pharmaceutical Society of Great Britain.

Karlsson, G. and Johannesson, M. (1996) 'The decision rules of cost-effectiveness analysis', *PharmacoEconomics*, 9: 113–120.

Kind, P., Hardman, G. and Macran, S. (1999) *UK population norms for EQ-5D*, University of York, Centre for Health Economics, Discussion Paper 172.

National Institute for Clinical Excellence (NICE) (2004) *Guide to the methods of technology assessment.* London, NICE.

NHS Executive (2004) *Trust financial returns.* Leeds, NHS Executive.

Serruys, P. W., Unger, F., Sousa, J. E., Jatine, A., Bonnier, H. J. R. M., Schonberger, J. P. A. M. and *et al.* (2001) 'Comparison of coronary artery bypass surgery and stenting for the treatment of multivessel disease', *New England Journal of Medicine*, 344: 1117–1124.

Stinnett, A. A. and Mullahy, J. (1998) 'Net health benefits: a new framework for the analysis of uncertainty in cost-effectiveness analysis', *Medical Decision Making*, 18 (Suppl): S68–S80.

Stinnett, A. A. and Paltiel, A. D. (1997) 'Estimating CE ratios under second-order uncertainty: the mean ratio versus the ratio of means', *Medical Decision Making*, 17: 483–489.

Tambour, M., Zethraeus, N. and Johannesson, M. (1998) 'A note on confidence intervals in cost-effectiveness analysis', *International Journal of Technology Assessment in Health Care*, 14: 467–471.

The EUROPA investigators (2003) 'Efficacy of perindopril in reduction of cardiovascular events among patients with stable coronary artery disease: randomised, double-blind, placebo-controlled, multicentre trial (the EUROPA study)', *Lancet*, 362: 782–788.

van Hout, B., Al, M. J., Gordon, G. S. and Rutten, F. F. (1994) 'Costs, effects and C/E-ratios alongside a clinical trial', *Health Economics*, 3: 309–319.

Weinstein, M. C. and Fineberg, H. V. (1980) *Clinical decision analysis.* Philadelphia, PA, WB Saunders Company.

Chapter 6

Decision making, uncertainty and the value of information

In this chapter we discuss how the results of probabilistic decision modelling should be interpreted and how decisions should be made in the light of the type of analysis described in the previous chapters. We identify two decisions which must be made: (i) should a technology be adopted on the basis of existing evidence, and (ii) whether further evidence is required to support this decision in the future. The first decision is dealt with in the following section. Measures of value of information, which can inform the second decision are covered subsequently. The role of this type of analysis in identifying research priorities, including the results of two recent UK pilot studies are then presented, followed by exercises to take you through this type of analysis.

6.1. Decision making with uncertainty

In this section we discuss how the results of probabilistic decision modelling should be interpreted and how decisions should be made in the light of the type of analysis described in the previous chapters. In order to do so we must first identify the decisions faced by health care systems and then consider what type of decision rules will be consistent with both the objectives and the constraint of the health care system.

6.1.1. What are the decisions?

There are two conceptually distinct but simultaneous decisions that must be made within any health care system. Firstly, should a technology be adopted or reimbursed given the existing evidence and the current uncertainty surrounding outcomes and resource use? In particular, which of the range of possible strategies, some of which may use the technology in different ways (e.g. at different points in the sequence of patient management and have different starting and discontinuation criteria), should be adopted? This question must also be addressed for the range of possible patient groups based on characteristics that may be related to expected costs and outcome (e.g. baseline and competing risks, age, as well as those which may be related to relative effects of the interventions).

Secondly, is additional evidence required to support these adoption or reimbursement decisions? As well as deciding whether more evidence is required in general, it is also important to know what type of evidence (for particular uncertain parameters) would be most valuable; what design of studies would be most useful in generating the type of evidence required, and how much of this evidence is required. There is also a need to address what type and level of evidence may be required across the range of relevant patient groups. So, as well as addressing whether more evidence is required there is also a range of decisions about the appropriate design of any subsequent research.

By clearly distinguishing these two separate but related decisions in health technology assessment, it is possible to identify analytic methods that can inform the adoption decision, the decision to acquire more evidence and inform research design in a way which is consistent with the objective and constraints on health care provision. This is not possible using more traditional evaluation approaches based on hypothesis testing and levels of statistical significance which combine these separate decisions and consequently fail to provide an adequate guide to either.

Requirements for decision making

These policy decisions indicate a number of requirements that an analytic framework must meet. These include a clear specification of the objectives and constraints of health care provision; a means of structuring the decision problem; a characterization of the uncertainty surrounding the decision; and a means of interpreting the results of the analysis so that decisions about adoption and additional evidence can be made in a way which is consistent with both the objectives and constraints on health care provision.

6.1.2. **A framework for analysis**

Bayesian decision theory and value of information analysis provides an analytic framework which can address whether a technology should be adopted based on current evidence and whether more evidence is required to support this decision in the future (Claxton *et al.* 2002). These methods have firm foundations in statistical decision theory (Raiffa and Schlaifer 1959; Pratt *et al.* 1995) and have been successfully used in other areas of research, such as engineering and environmental risk analysis (Howard 1966; Thompson and Evans 1997). More recently these methods have been extended to setting priorities in the evaluation of health care technologies (Claxton and Posnett 1996; Claxton 1999*a*; Claxton *et al.* 2002). In addition, they have been usefully applied to a number of different health technologies (Yokota and Thompson 2004; Ginnelly *et al.* 2005), and have been piloted as a means of setting research priorities for the UK NHS and informing the National Institute for Clinical Excellence (NICE) in making research recommendations (Claxton *et al.* 2004; Claxton *et al.* 2005*a*).

The application of these methods requires three core tasks to be completed: (i) the construction of a decision analytic model to represent the decision problem; (ii) a probabilistic analysis of this model to characterize the current decision uncertainty; and (iii) establishing the value of additional information. The first two tasks have been dealt with in previous chapters. In this chapter we address how the results of probabilistic modelling should be interpreted by decision makers and how to address the question of whether more evidence is required.

As we saw at the end of Chapter 5, the uncertainty surrounding the decision problem can be characterized by 'propagating' these distributions through the model using Monte Carlo simulation methods. The output of these simulations provides the joint distribution of expected costs and outcomes for each strategy being compared. The uncertainty surrounding the cost-effectiveness of a technology, for a range of thresholds for cost-effectiveness, can be represented as a cost-effectiveness acceptability curve (CEAC). Figure 6.1 illustrates an example of a CEAC for a simple model of zanamivir for the treatment of influenza.

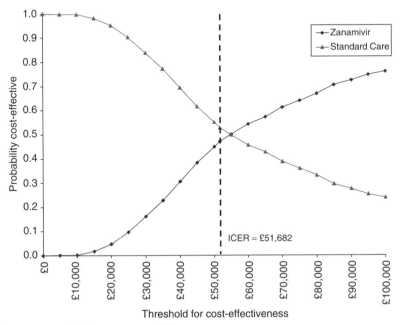

Fig. 6.1 Cost-effectiveness acceptability curve.

This is a probabilistic reanalysis of the model contained in the independent Technology Assessment Report, which was submitted as part of the NICE appraisal of zanamivir in 2000 (Burles *et al.* 2000; NICE 2000). In this example, the probability that the intervention is cost-effective increases as the willingness to pay for additional health (quality-adjusted life-years) or the threshold for cost-effectiveness increases. The incremental cost-effectiveness ratio, based on expected incremental costs and incremental QALYs, is £51 682. Thus, if the threshold for cost-effectiveness was just greater than £51 682, then the intervention could be regarded as cost-effective, even though the probability that it is cost-effective is less than 0.5 (0.472). This is because the distribution of the additional net benefits is positively skewed, with a mean greater than its median value. The decision uncertainty can be represented by including a cost-effectiveness frontier (Fenwick *et al.* 2001). As discussed in Chapter 5, the frontier indicates the probability that the alternative with the highest net-benefit will be cost-effective. The decision uncertainty or the error probability is then 1 minus the value of the frontier.

The question is how should this be interpreted by decision makers and how should the decision be made under uncertainty? For example, if society was willing to pay £60 000 per QALY gained then the probability that zanamivir is cost-effective is only 0.52 and the error probability is therefore 0.48. In these circumstances, what decision should be made about zanamivir?

6.1.3. **The irrelevance of inference**

If we base decisions on the traditional rules of inference (either frequentist or Bayesian) then we would conclude that the apparent cost-effectiveness of zanamivir is not statistically significant or falls within a Bayesian range of equivalence; we cannot reject the null hypothesis and the result is indeterminate. In practice this would lead to the rejection of zanamivir, despite the fact that it is the alternative with the highest probability of being cost-effective and, more importantly, has the highest expected net-benefit on the basis of the information currently available. If we fail to adopt an intervention simply because the differences in net-benefit are not regarded as statistically significant or the error probability is 'too high' then we will impose opportunity costs on patients who could benefit from it. These opportunity costs are the forgone expected net benefits resulting from selecting a technology with a lower expected net-benefit. For an individual patient in the zanamivir example, these forgone expected net benefits are £3.07 or 0.000052 QALYs at a cost-effectiveness threshold of £60 000. For the UK population of current and future patients they could be valued at £2 748 276 or 45.8 QALYs

If the objective underlying health technology assessment is to make decisions that are consistent with maximizing health gains from available resources, then decisions should be based on expected cost-effectiveness (net-benefit) given the existing information. This is irrespective of whether any differences are regarded as statistically significant or fall outside a Bayesian range of equivalence. The traditional rules of inference impose unnecessary costs on individual patients and on the population of current and future patients and are irrelevant to the choice between alternative technologies (Claxton 1999*b*).

This is because one of the (mutually exclusive) alternatives must be chosen and this decision cannot be deferred. For example, by rejecting the new technology we are selecting current practice and vice versa. The opportunity cost of failing to make the correct decision based on expectation is symmetrical and the historical accident that dictates which of the alternatives is regarded as 'current practice' is irrelevant. No one would ever suggest that a new treatment should be adopted when its mean net-benefit is less than current practice but, in terms of opportunity cost, this is precisely what is implied by the arbitrary rules of inference.

Of course, the measure of net-benefit is based on a particular objective (maximize health outcomes) or social welfare function which may be judged inappropriate, and consequently, this measure may be regarded as incomplete. However, if there are equity issues that need to be incorporated, they can be made explicit with appropriate adjustments to the measure of outcome. Similarly, if there is particular concern for safety and rare but catastrophic events, then these undesirable outcomes should be given appropriate weight in the calculation of expected net benefits. If decision makers wish to adopt some type of voting rule, then the decision may focus on the median rather than the mean net benefits, and the treatment which benefits the greatest number could be adopted. Attitudes to risk can be incorporated in the measures of outcome, and if we wish to incorporate the fact that some individuals' preferences violate the axioms of expected utility theory, then prospect theory or some notion of regret can be used in the measure of net benefits. It is not necessary to take a position on the appropriate social welfare function, different definitions of need, the normative content of expected utility theory, or the best way to incorporate important and legitimate equity concerns to accept the irrelevance of inference. It is worth noting, however, that these considerations will all have implications for the measures of outcome and the design of studies, not just their interpretation. Whatever view is taken, confidence intervals, *P*-values and levels of significance still remain entirely irrelevant to the decision.

6.2. **Expected value of perfect information**

Although decisions should be based on expected cost-effectiveness given the existing information, this does not mean that adoption decisions can simply be based on little, or poor quality, evidence, as long as the decision to conduct further research to support adoption (or rejection) is made simultaneously.

Decisions based on existing information will be uncertain, and there will always be a chance that the 'wrong' decision will be made. That is, although we make the correct decision now based on our current estimate of expected net-benefit, there is a chance that another alternative would have had higher net-benefit once our current uncertainties are resolved. If our decision based on current information turns out to be 'wrong', there will be costs in terms of health benefit and resources forgone. Therefore, the expected cost of uncertainty is determined jointly by the probability that a decision based on existing information will be wrong and the consequences of a wrong decision. With estimates of the probability of error and the opportunity costs of error we can calculate the expected cost of uncertainty or the expected opportunity loss surrounding the decisions. The expected costs of uncertainty can be interpreted as the expected value of perfect information (EVPI), as perfect information can eliminate the possibility of making the wrong decision. If the objective of the health care system is to maximize gains in health outcome subject to a budget constraint, then this is also the maximum that the health care system should be willing to pay for additional evidence to inform this decision in the future, and it places an upper bound on the value of conducting further research. If there are other objectives of health care provision, such as equity, which can be identified and valued, then these can be incorporated into the analysis and the societal value of information derived.

This general idea is illustrated in Fig. 6.2 for the choice between two alternatives. Three things determine the value of information. Firstly, how cost-effective (or ineffective) the technology appears given current or prior information (O'Hagan and Luce 2003), that is, the position of the expected (prior) incremental net-benefit that is valued in terms of health in Fig.6.2. Secondly, the uncertainty surrounding cost-effectiveness (or cost-ineffectiveness), that is, the distribution of the prior mean incremental net-benefit. Thirdly, the slope of the loss function which values the consequences of decision error based on current information. In Fig. 6.2a the expected incremental net-benefit is positive, so the new technology appears to be cost-effective given existing information. However, this decision is uncertain, and there is a probability of error represented by the tail area where incremental net-benefit is less than zero. If this is the way our current uncertainties resolve then it would have

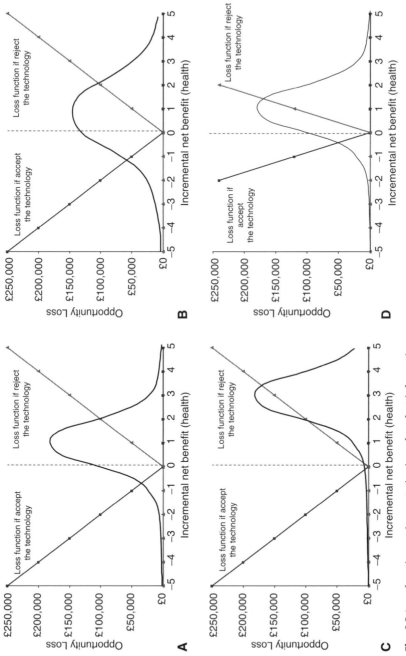

Fig. 6.2 Loss function and expected value of perfect information.

been better to reject the technology and there will be opportunity losses in the form of net-benefit forgone. These opportunity losses are represented by the loss function, which has a slope equal to the cost-effectiveness threshold and simply converts the incremental net-benefit measured in health terms on the X-axis into monetary terms on the Y-axis.

For example, in Fig. 6.2a it is possible that our decision based on expected incremental net benefits will be wrong, as there is a probability that the incremental net-benefit will be less than zero. If it is, then the cost of this error or the opportunity loss is the difference between the net-benefit we could have gained by making the right decision in these circumstances (reject the new technology) and the net-benefit we get from the decision based on the expected incremental net-benefit. This is represented by the height of the loss function and illustrates that there is a small chance that incremental net-benefit will be a lot less than zero (−5 QALY), in which case the opportunity loss will be very high (£250 000). However, there is a greater chance that the incremental net-benefit will be just less than zero (−1 QALY), in which case the opportunity loss will be lower (£50 000). The expected opportunity loss (EVPI) is essentially taking a weighted mean of all these losses where the weights are the probability of incurring each of these losses.

Figure 6.2b illustrates that where there is more uncertainty (greater variance in incremental net-benefit) then the probability of error (tail area) will increase and expected opportunity loss and, therefore, EVPI will be higher. In Fig. 6.2c the technology appears to be more cost-effective (mean of the distribution is further to the right), the probability of error falls and EVPI also falls; the technology appears so cost-effective there is little uncertainty about its adoption. In Fig. 6.2d the cost-effectiveness threshold is higher (the slope of the loss function is greater), opportunity losses (in health terms) are valued more highly and this will tend to increase the EVPI. However, increasing the cost-effectiveness threshold will also increase the expected incremental net-benefit (the distribution will shift to the right) and the probability of error will fall, therefore, the EVPI may fall. Figure 6.2 also indicates that the shape of the distribution also matters. In this case, with positive expected incremental net-benefit, if it was negatively skewed but with the same variance, there would be a higher chance of larger errors with greater opportunity loss and higher EVPI.

6.2.1. **EVPI using the normal distribution**

If incremental net-benefit can be regarded as normally distributed, then simple analytic solutions can be used to establish the EVPI surrounding the decision. The discussion of Fig. 6.2 provides some intuition when considering these analytic solutions, which have been used in the earlier literature on value-of-information analysis (Raiffa and Schlaifer 1959; Claxton and Posnett 1996). Each of the three issues discussed in the previous section are represented in the expression for EVPI:

$$\text{EVPI} = \lambda \cdot \sigma_0 \cdot L(D_0),$$

where:

λ = cost-effectiveness threshold
$D_0 = |\eta_0|/\sigma_0$
η_0 = prior mean incremental net health benefit
σ_0^2 = prior variance of the incremental net-benefit (η_0)
$L(D_0)$ = unit normal loss integral for D_0

The unit normal loss integral is the integration of a loss function with slope of 1 with a standard normal distribution (mean = 0 and $\sigma_0 = 1$). Therefore, $L(D_0)$ represents probability of decision error when incremental net-benefit has a mean of D_0 and $\sigma_0 = 1$. The probability of decision error is determined by: (i) the standardized distance (D_0) of the prior mean incremental net benefits of the technology (η_0) from the point at which the decision based on current information would switch (where $\eta_0 = 0$), that is, how cost-effective the technology appears to be; and (ii) the uncertainty surrounding η_0 (Var(η_0) = σ_0^2). The slope of the loss function is the cost-effectiveness threshold (λ) and represents the monetary value placed on opportunity losses when they are incurred. So, this expression for the EVPI reflects the determinants of the probability of error and the consequences of error illustrated in Fig. 6.2.

You will find this approach taken in earlier papers on value-of-information analysis (Claxton and Posnett 1996, Claxton 1999a, Claxton et al. 2001). It will be appropriate if incremental net-benefit is normally distributed. This may be the case if all the evidence for costs and benefits comes from the same sample, in which case central limit theorem may assure normality. However, decision models combine evidence from a variety of sources and, as discussed in Chapter 4, use a range of distributions assigned to parameters. The resulting net-benefit from probabilistic analysis is a mixture of these distributions, through a model structure which is likely to be nonlinear and may contain discontinuities generated by logical functions. In addition, there may be complex correlation structures generated between parameter estimates when evidence is synthesized. In these circumstances there is no reason to believe that net-benefit will be normally distributed. In fact, it is unlikely to have a parametric distribution at all. Therefore, a nonparametric approach to establishing EVPI is required. This type of approach is outlined in the next section and is now most commonly used in the evaluation of health technologies.

6.2.1. **Nonparametric approach to EVPI**

We do not need to be restricted to analytic solutions that require assumptions of normality because we can work out the EVPI directly from the simulated output from our model. With current information, decisions must be made before we know how the uncertainties will be resolved, that is, we must make a decision now based on the expected net benefits of each of the alternatives. However, with perfect information, we could make our decisions once we know how the uncertainties in the model will resolve, so we could make different decisions for different resolutions of net-benefit. The EVPI is simply the difference between the payoff (expected net-benefit) with perfect and current information (Pratt *et al.* 1995; Thompson and Graham 1996; Felli and Hazen 1998; Ades *et al.* 2004; Sculpher and Claxton 2005).

For example, if there are *j* alternative interventions, with unknown parameters θ, then given the existing evidence, the optimal decision is the intervention that generates the maximum expected net-benefit:

$$\max_j E_\theta NB(j, \theta),$$

that is, choose *j* with the maximum net benefits over all the iterations from the simulation because each iteration represents a possible future realization of the existing uncertainty (a possible value of θ). With perfect information, the decision maker would know how the uncertainties would resolve (which value θ will take) before making a decision and could select the intervention that maximizes the net-benefit given a particular value of θ:

$$\max_j NB(j, \theta).$$

However, the true values of θ are unknown (we don't know in advance which value θ will take). Therefore, the expected value of a decision taken with perfect information is found by averaging the maximum net-benefit over the joint distribution of θ:

$$E_\theta \max_j NB(j, \theta).$$

In other words, first calculate the maximum net-benefit for each iteration from the simulation (for a particular value of θ), then take the mean over these maximum net benefits (over the possible values of θ). The expected value of perfect information for an individual patient is simply the difference between the expected value of the decision made with perfect information about the uncertain parameters θ, and the decision made on the basis of existing evidence:

$$\text{EVPI} = E_\theta \max_j NB(j, \theta) - \max_j E_\theta NB(j, \theta).$$

Table 6.1 Calculating EVPI

	Treatment A	B	Optimal choice	Maximum net-benefit	Opportunity loss
Iteration 1	9	12	B	12	0
Iteration 2	12	10	A	12	2
Iteration 3	14	20	B	20	0
Iteration 4	11	10	A	11	1
Iteration 5	14	13	A	14	1
Expectation	12	13		13.8	0.8

This approach is illustrated in Table 6.1 for two alternative treatments A and B. The table represents simulated output from five iterations generating a net-benefit for each of the treatments. With current information, the best a decision maker can do is to choose the alternative with the highest expected net-benefit ($\max_j E_\theta NB(j, \theta)$) which, in this case, is to choose treatment B with expected net-benefit of 13. With perfect information the decision maker could choose the alternative with the maximum net-benefit (columns 3 and 4) for each resolution of uncertainty ($\max_j NB(j, \theta)$), that is, choose B for iteration 1; A for iteration 2 and B for iteration 3 etc. However, we do not know in advance which of these possibilities will turn out to be true, so the expected net-benefit with perfect information is simply the expectation of the maximum net-benefit (£13.80). The EVPI is then simply the difference between the expected net-benefit with perfect information and the expected net-benefit with current information (£13.80 − £13.00 = £0.80). This is entirely equivalent to taking the expectation of the opportunity losses in column 5, where opportunity loss is simply the difference between the net-benefit of optimal choice for that iteration and the alternative that would be chosen based on current information. This confirms the earlier discussion that EVPI is also the expected opportunity loss or the expected costs of the uncertainty surrounding the decision. It should be noted that in this example, although alternative B has the highest expected net-benefit, it also has a lower probability of being cost-effective ($P = 0.4$) than alternative A ($P = 0.6$), demonstrating the importance of cost-effectiveness frontiers as discussed in Chapter 5.

This provides the EVPI surrounding the decision as a whole for each time this decision is made (for an individual patient or individual patient episode). However, once information is generated to inform the decision for an individual patient or patient episode then it is also available to inform the management of all other current and future patients (it has public good characteristics and is nonrival). Therefore, it is important that EVPI is expressed for the total population of patients who stand to benefit from additional information over the expected lifetime of the technology. This requires some assessment of the effective lifetime of the technology, the period over which information about the decision will be useful (T), and estimates of incidence over this period (I_t).

$$\text{EVPI for the population} \;=\; \text{EVPI}. \Sigma_{t=1, 2, \dots, T}\, I_t / (1+r)^t.$$

The EVPI associated with future patients is discounted at rate r to provide the total EVPI for the population of current and future patients (see Chapter 7 for further discussion of this issue).

Figure 6.3 illustrates the population EVPI for the example used in Fig. 6.1. If this population EVPI exceeds the expected costs of additional research, then it is potentially cost-effective to conduct further research. For example, if additional research is expected to cost £1m then additional research is *potentially* cost-effective if the threshold is greater than £31 000 per QALY. At lower values of the threshold, the new technology should be rejected based on current evidence and further research is required to support this decision because the returns from further research cannot offset the costs.

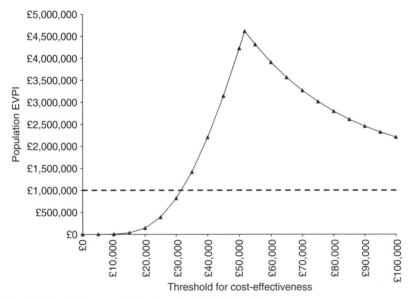

Fig. 6.3 Population expected value of perfect information curve.

The relationship between the EVPI and the cost-effectiveness threshold in Fig. 6.3 has an intuitive interpretation. When the threshold for cost-effectiveness is low, the technology is not expected to be cost-effective and additional information is unlikely to change that decision (EVPI is low). Thus, current evidence can be regarded as sufficient to support the decision to reject the technology. In these circumstances the EVPI increases with the threshold because the decision uncertainty (probability of error) increases and the consequences of decision error (opportunity loss) are valued more highly. Conversely, when the threshold is higher than the incremental cost-effectiveness ratio (ICER), the intervention is expected to be cost-effective and this decision is less likely to be changed by further research as the threshold is increased. The decision uncertainty falls because the technology appears to be increasingly cost-effective as the threshold is increased (probability of error falls, tending to reduce the EVPI), but the consequences of error are valued more highly (tending to increase the EVPI). In this example the reduction in decision uncertainty offsets the increased value of the consequences of error. However, the EVPI will ultimately increase with very high values of the threshold because the decision uncertainty falls at a declining rate, but the value of opportunity losses increases at a constant rate and will ultimately offset this. In this particular example, the population EVPI reaches a maximum when the threshold is equal to the expected incremental cost-effectiveness ratio of this technology. In other words, in this case the EVPI reaches a maximum when we are most uncertain about whether to adopt or reject the technology based on existing evidence.

The EVPI curve for two alternatives is easy to interpret. However, most decision problems involve more than two alternatives. The principles of calculating EVPI remain the same (see the section on EVPI for strategies later in this chapter) but the EVPI curve can take a variety of shapes depending on whether the alternatives being considered are cost-effective at some value of the threshold (in which case there will be a number of peaks or changes in the slope of the EVPI curve at threshold values equal to the ICER of each of the alternatives), or if some of the alternatives are dominated or extendedly dominated (the peak or discontinuity will be in negative threshold space: we would only wish to adopt the alternative if we were willing to pay to *reduce* health outcome).

It should be clear from this discussion of EVPI that the value of further research will depend on both the uncertainty surrounding estimates of cost and effect but also on how cost-effective or cost-ineffective a technology is expected to be, given existing evidence and the size of the patient population that could benefit from additional research. One implication is that it is perfectly possible that the value of additional evidence about a new technology, which is substantially cost-effective based on existing evidence, will be very low even if there is uncertainty surrounding the parameters. That is, there may be uncertainty in cost and outcomes, but the decision uncertainty – and therefore the EVPI – may still be low. In these circumstances, the technology should be adopted and no further research is required to support this decision.

This discussion of value-of-information analysis suggests that there will be different values of information for different technologies applied to different patient populations and for the same technology in different circumstances, such as for different indications, patient populations and in different health care systems with different cost-effectiveness thresholds. This is illustrated in Fig. 6.4 which shows the EVPI associated with five stylized examples of health care technologies, which were appraised by NICE between 1999 and 2000. It shows that we should demand different amounts of evidence for different technologies and that there can be no fixed rules for regulatory or reimbursement decisions (Claxton 1999b). How much evidence is required to support a decision is essentially an empirical question. Figure 6.4 also illustrates the difference between parameter and decision uncertainty. For example, the prophylactic extraction of wisdom teeth (WT) has the most parameter uncertainty (there was very little and poor quality evidence). However, there is no

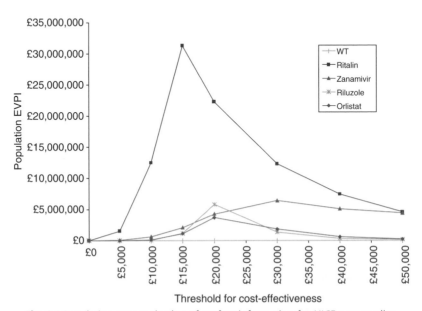

Fig. 6.4 Population expected value of perfect information for NICE case studies.

decision uncertainty and no value of information because there is very little doubt that this is not cost-effective, despite the uncertainty in costs and outcomes.

Of course, there is no such thing as perfect information but it does place an upper bound on the returns to research. The population EVPI can be used as a first hurdle to identify research that is potentially cost-effective and rule out research which will not be worthwhile. However, we should be cautious when comparing EVPI across technologies as in Fig. 6.4. This is because the cost of research may differ and the marginal benefits of actual research may also differ across these technologies.

The framework of analysis, which has been outlined above allows us to take a rational approach to decision making with uncertainty. By separating the two questions of whether to adopt a technology given existing information from the question of whether more information is needed to inform this choice in the future, we can get sensible answers to both. As EVPI is so easy to establish directly from the simulation once a probabilistic model has been developed, there is no reason why decision EVPI should not be a routine part of any evaluation.

6.3. Expected value of perfect information for parameters

The EVPI surrounding the decision problem can indicate whether further research is potentially worthwhile. However, it would be useful to have an indication of what type of additional evidence would be most valuable. In Chapter 5 we introduced ANCOVA as a measure of the importance of a parameter. As was noted, however, these rely on linearity, are not directly related to decision uncertainty, and cannot provide a measure of value that can be compared with the costs of further investigation. The value of reducing the uncertainty surrounding particular parameters in the decision model can be established using a similar approach to the EVPI for the decision problem as a whole. This type of analysis can be used to focus research on the type of evidence that will be most important by identifying those parameters for which more precise estimates would be most valuable. In some circumstances, this will indicate which endpoints should be included in further experimental research. In other circumstances, it may focus research on getting more precise estimates of particular parameters that may not necessarily require experimental design and may be provided relatively quickly. The analysis of the value of information associated with each of the model inputs is, in principle, conducted in a very similar way to the EVPI for the decision as a whole (Pratt *et al.* 1995; Thompson and Evans 1997; Ades *et al.* 2004).

The expected value of perfect information for a parameter(s) (EVPPI) is simply the difference between the expected value with perfect and current information about the parameter(s). The expected value with perfect information is found by taking the maximum expected net-benefit given perfect information only about the parameter(s) of interest (calculating expected net benefits over all the other uncertain parameters in the model) and then calculating the mean of all the possible values of the parameter of interest. The EVPI for the parameter is simply the difference between the expected net-benefit with perfect information and the expected value with current information (the same as for decision EVPI). However, this does require substantial additional computation for models where the relationship between the parameters and the expected cost and outcomes is not linear, for example in Markov models.

More formally, suppose we were interested in the value of perfect information about a parameter or a subset (φ) of all the uncertain parameters θ. With perfect information we would know how φ would resolve (which value it will take) and the expected net-benefit of a decision would be found by choosing the alternative with the maximum expected net-benefit when those expected net benefits are averaged over the remaining uncertain parameters in the model (ψ). In other words, we take a value of φ and then calculate expected net benefits over the remaining uncertainties (ψ) and choose the alternative j that has the maximum expected net-benefit:

$$\max_j E_{\psi|\varphi} \, NB(\, j, \, \varphi, \psi).$$

As before, however, the true values of φ are unknown (we do not know what value φ will take), therefore, the expected value of a decision taken with perfect information is found by averaging the maximum expected net benefits over the distribution of φ:

$$E_\varphi \max_j E_{\psi|\varphi} NB(\, j, \, \varphi, \psi).$$

The expected value with current information is the same as before because $\varphi \cup \psi = \theta$):

$$\max_j E_\theta NB(\, j, \, \theta).$$

So the EVPPI for the parameter or group of parameters φ is simply the difference between the expected value of a decision made with perfect information and the expected value with current information:

$$\text{EVPPI}_\varphi \; = \; E_\varphi \max_j E_{\psi|\varphi} NB(\, j, \, \varphi, \psi) \, - \, \max_j E_\theta NB(\, j, \, \theta).$$

It should be apparent that although this is conceptually very similar to the initially discussed calculation for decision EVPI, it is also more computationally intensive. This is because we have an inner and outer loop of expectation: first we must run the simulation for parameters ψ but with a particular value of φ (an inner loop), then we must sample a new value of φ (an outer loop) and rerun the simulation. This must be repeated until we have sampled sufficiently from the distribution (or joint distribution) of φ.

This suggests that when choosing how many iterations to run on the inner and outer loops, as you will do in the exercise, there is no reason why we should choose an equal number of iterations. Although there can be no clear rules, it seems reasonable that we will need more iterations when there are more uncertain parameters in order to sample from the whole of the joint distribution. For example, if φ is only one parameter and ψ contains, say, 20 parameters, then it makes more sense to run more iterations on the inner than the outer loop. However, there are many circumstances where we will want to calculate the EVPPI for groups of parameters together. In this case there may be ten parameters in ψ and ten in φ. In this case an equal number of simulations in the inner and outer loop would seem more reasonable.

One implication of this discussion is that, just as with decision uncertainty, information about a parameter is only valuable if it is possible for it to change the decision (which alternative has the maximum expected net-benefit). Therefore, information is only valuable insofar as uncertain parameters do not resolve at their expected value. This suggests that those parameters that are more uncertain (can resolve at extreme values) *and* are closely related to *differences* in net-benefit between the alternatives, are likely to have a greater value of information associated with them. However, parameters that may be very uncertain but have little effect on the *differences* in net-benefit (e.g. changes the cost or the effects of each alternative to an equal extent or in way that offsets each other) may have a very low or even zero EVPPI. This, as well as the issues raised in the next two paragraphs, sometimes makes it very difficult to 'guess' which parameters or groups of parameters will have high EVPPI associated with them in anything but the simplest of models. Of course, counter-intuitive results should prompt careful scrutiny of the model and the analysis to understand the results. However, we should take no comfort from what appear to be intuitive results, because if it really were that easy then there would be no point in building a model.

6.3.1. **Groups of parameters**

It is very important to recognise that the EVPPI for the individual parameters do not sum to the decision EVPI. Equally, the EVPPI for a group of parameters is not the sum of the individual parameter EVPPIs. This is because the individual parameters when considered in isolation may not resolve in such a way as to have a sufficient impact on differences in net-benefit to change the decision. However, when a group of parameters is considered together, then the joint effect of each resolving at an extreme value may have sufficient impact on differences in net-benefit to change the decision and generate a value of information. It is perfectly possible that the EVPPI for all the individual parameters may be zero, but for the decision and for groups of parameters it may be substantial.

This discussion indicates that it is best to approach EVPPI analysis by initially conducting EVPPI analysis on a small number of groups of parameters. The groups should be chosen to match the type of research that would be conducted. For example, it would be reasonable to group all the parameters that may be vulnerable to selection bias and would require randomized design. It would also make sense to group all those parameters associated with natural history or baseline risk, which may be informed by observational or epidemiological studies, and group all those associated with quality of life that could be informed by a survey. Then, if there is significant EVPPI associated with a group of parameters, it can then be broken down by conducting EVPPI on smaller groups or individual parameters to identify where the value of information lies. This is much more efficient than starting with EVPPI for all parameters and then combining them in different ways. More importantly it is much more relevant to informing decisions about research priorities.

Another important reason to group parameters is if they are correlated. The EVPPI for the groups of correlated parameters will preserve the correlation structure. However, conducting EVPPI in the way described above on only one of the correlated parameters will break this correlation. The EVPPI could either be under-or overestimated depending on the type correlation between the parameters, the direction of the relationship of each parameter to differences in net-benefit, and the decision based on current information. Where there is correlation between parameters it is also possible for the EVPPI on one of the correlated parameters to be greater than the EVPI for the group of correlated parameters and in some circumstances greater than the decision EVPI.

6.3.2. **EVPPI for linear models**

The approach to EVPPI outlined above provides a general solution for non-linear models. However, it is also more computationally intensive because it requires an inner and outer loop of simulation. The computational requirements can be somewhat simplified if the model has either a linear or multilinear relationship between the parameters and net-benefit. If the model is linear in ψ, and φ and ψ are independent then:

$$E_{\psi|\varphi}NB(j,\varphi,\psi) \;=\; NB(j, \varphi,E(\psi)).$$

The expected net-benefit for a particular value of φ can be calculated based on the mean values of the other parameters ψ, and the inner loop of simulation is unnecessary. This will also be true when net-benefit is multilinear in ψ and where there are no correlations between the parameters in ψ and when φ and ψ are also independent. Multilinearity allows the net-benefit function to contain products of (independent) parameters. This 'short cut' may, therefore, be used for many standard decision tree models, with branching path probabilities and independent parameters (Felli and Hazen 1998; Ades *et al.* 2004).

Reduction in opportunity loss

In Table 6.1 we demonstrated that EVPI was also the expected opportunity loss or the expected cost of uncertainty. It is natural to interpret EVPPI as the reduction in opportunity loss or the reduction in the cost of uncertainty if we had perfect information about the parameters of interest. In other words it is the difference between the decision EVPI and the EVPI for the decision when we have perfect information about the parameters of interest. This is true as long as we calculate the EVPI for the decision over all the ways the parameter can resolve and not simply its expected value. It can easily be shown that the terms in these expressions cancel and this approach does lead (in the limit and without spurious correlation) to the EVPPI outlined above. It is consistent with the well-known identity of maximizing expected value (net-benefit) and minimizing opportunity loss. Although this approach has been taken in the past, the approach set out above is recommended as it is easier to implement and avoids unnecessary noise and spurious correlation in the simulation.

6.3.3. **EVPI for multiple treatment options**

The initially discussed requirements for decision making included the estimation of the expected costs and health outcomes for each of the possible strategies that could be adopted, including the range of possible strategies (not just those directly compared in current trial evidence), and for a range of clinical policies (how a technology could be used). The inclusion of all possible alternatives or strategies within the analysis is necessary to inform the adoption decision but it is also crucial for the estimation of the value of information.

Even when an alternative is never regarded as cost-effective over a range of possible threshold values, due to dominance or extended dominance, there may be a chance that it could be cost-effective. Indeed, an alternative which is regarded as dominated or extendedly dominated may have a higher chance of being cost-effective at a particular threshold value than an alternative which is not dominated (Claxton and Thompson 2001). In these circumstances, excluding the alternative from the analysis may not change the decision about which strategy should be regarded as cost-effective based on current information, but it will have a substantial impact on the EVPI. Indeed, the exclusion of any strategy from the analysis will reduce the decision EVPI if there is a non-zero probability that it could be cost-effective, because there may be particular resolutions of the uncertain parameters where the excluded strategy would provide the maximum net-benefit.

The principles of calculating EVPI for multiple alternatives remains the same as was illustrated in Table 6.1 for the choice between two alternatives A and B. Table 6.2 illustrates how to calculate the EVPI when alternatives C and D are also available.

As before, the table represents simulated output from five iterations, generating net benefits for each of the now four strategies. With current information, the alternative with the highest expected net-benefit remains B with an expected net-benefit of 13. With perfect information, the decision maker can choose the alternative with the maximum net-benefit, which will now be alternative C for iterations 1 and 4. Therefore, the expected net-benefit with perfect information (the expectation of the maximum net benefits) has increased from £13.80 to £14.40 and the EVPI has increased from £0.80 to £1.40. So, although alternative C is not cost-effective based on current information, there is a chance that it will be. Excluding C will not effect the decision to adopt B but it may affect the decision to conduct further research. Alternative D, on the other hand, is never the optimal choice in these five iterations (there is no chance that it will be cost-effective) and its inclusion or exclusion has no effect on the EVPI.

Table 6.2 Calculating EVPI for multiple alternatives

	A	B	C	D	Optimal choice	Maximum net-benefit	Opportunity loss
Iteration 1	9	12	14	8	C	14	2
Iteration 2	12	10	8	7	A	12	2
Iteration 3	14	20	15	12	B	20	0
Iteration 4	11	10	12	9	C	12	2
Iteration 5	14	13	11	10	A	14	1
Expectation	12	13	12	9		14.4	1.4

The difference between the EVPI for the full decision problem (all strategies) and the EVPI when a strategy is excluded from the analysis can indicate the bias in EVPI that is introduced by excluding the strategy. For example, excluding C from the analysis would lead to the EVPI being underestimated by £0.60. However, this difference in EVPI should not be interpreted as the EVPI associated with the strategy. This is for two reasons: (i) this difference conflates the value of the strategy itself (improvement in net-benefit) and its contribution to decision uncertainty; and (ii) many model parameters are relevant to more than one strategy. The only meaningful measure is the value of information associated with those parameters that are specific to the strategy, such as the relative effectiveness of a technology that is specific to the strategy.

It is possible to use value-of-information analysis to decide whether a strategy should be included as relevant or can be safely excluded from the analysis. For example, in Table 6.2, if after 10 000 iterations, D was still never optimal (the probability it is cost-effective is effectively zero) then it could be safely excluded from further analysis because its exclusion has no effect on the EVPI. In this sense, we can use value of information to define relevant comparators and exclude others, that is, any strategy is potentially a relevant comparator if it has some chance of being cost-effective and therefore contributes to the EVPI. However, to decide whether particular strategies that contribute to EVPI should be compared in subsequent research requires measures of value-of-sample information; this is discussed in Chapter 8 (Claxton and Thompson 2001). It should be noted that what is and what is not relevant will depend on the particular value of the cost-effectiveness threshold.

6.3.4. **An example of EVPPI**

Figure 6.5 illustrates the EVPPIs associated with the decision EVPI in Fig. 6.3 at a threshold of £40 000 per QALY. In this example, the EVPPI associated with reduction in symptom days on zanamivir is relatively high. A more precise estimate of the reduction in symptom days will require experimental design to avoid selection bias and suggests that further randomized trials may be worthwhile. However, other parameters with lower EVPPI such as the quality of life associated with influenza symptoms (QALY/day); the probability of hospitalization with standard care (P(hospitalization)); and the probability that a patient presenting with influenza-like symptoms does in fact have influenza (P(disease)) may not require experimental research and may be important if the costs of further investigation (resources and delay) are low. Other parameters such as the probability of complications requiring antibiotics with standard care (P(complications)) have negligible EVPPI and are relatively unimportant. The impact of zanamivir on complications requiring

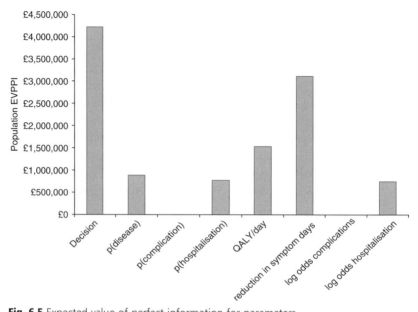

Fig. 6.5 Expected value of perfect information for parameters.

antibiotics (log odds ratio (complications)) has negligible EVPPI but the impact on hospitalization (log odds ratio (hospitalization)) has positive EVPPI. This suggests that if a trial is conducted to provide a more precise estimate of the reduction in symptom days then also measuring the impact on hospitalizations could be worthwhile. It is clear in Fig. 6.5 that the EVPPIs will not necessarily sum to the overall decision EVPI for the reasons outlined above.

Figure 6.6 illustrates the relationship between EVPPI for the model parameters and the cost-effectiveness threshold. The EVPPIs for the model parameters are related to the cost-effectiveness threshold in the same way as decision EVPI (illustrated in Fig. 6.3). In this example, just as with decision EVPI, the EVPPIs reach a maximum when the cost-effectiveness threshold is equal to the ICER for zanamivir, that is, when the prior mean incremental net-benefit is zero. At low cost-effectiveness thresholds (<£25 000) the EVPPI is negligible because zanamivir is not cost-effective at these values and standard care is chosen based on current information. In these circumstances, even if individual model parameters resolve at their extreme values, they are unlikely to change this decision. Clearly the absolute value of EVPPI changes with the threshold just as decision EVPI changes. However, the relative importance of each parameter (and the ranking) may also change with the cost-effectiveness threshold.

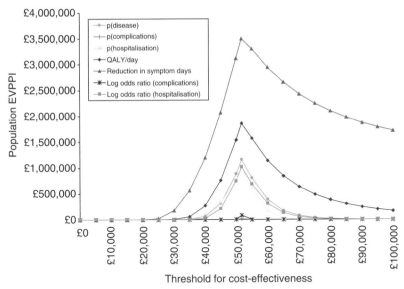

Fig. 6.6 Expected value of perfect information for parameters.

In general, those parameters that are more closely related to differences in costs will be more important at lower thresholds; those that are more closely related to differences in effect will be more important at higher threshold values. This demonstrates that the value of research and the type of research required depends on the threshold for cost-effectiveness. In other words, not only is the value of further research essentially an economic question, but the type and design of future research is an economic question too.

The earlier discussion of decision EVPI suggested that what might be regarded as sufficient evidence is an empirical question, which will differ across technologies and will depend on the cost-effectiveness threshold used in decision making, as well as the amount and quality of evidence available. This was illustrated using five stylised examples of health care technologies which were considered by NICE in Fig. 6.4. Figure 6.7 illustrates the EVPPI for these stylised examples, where parameters have been grouped into effect, utilities and cost. The EVPI associated with effect, utilities and cost differs across these technologies. For example, it is additional evidence about the relationship between clinical measures of effect and quality of life which is most valuable to inform the decisions to adopt Ritalin® for the treatment of ADHD and orlistat for the treatment of obesity. However, it is additional evidence about clinical effect which is most valuable when considering the use of zanamivir for the treatment of influenza, and additional evidence about the expected

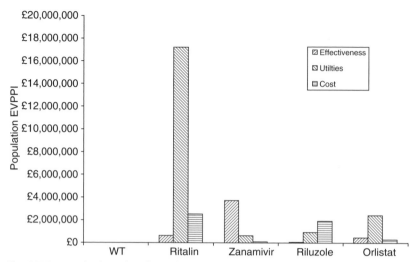

Fig. 6.7 Expected value of perfect information for parameters for the stylized NICE examples.

costs of motor neurone disease when considering the use of riluzole. This demonstrates that not only will we want different amounts of evidence for different technologies (and different amounts of the same technology but in different circumstances), we will also want different types of evidence. Again, there are clear implications for the efficient regulation and reimbursement of health technologies (Claxton 1999*b*).

In this section we have demonstrated that the value of information associated with individual parameters or groups of parameters can be established using the same principles as decision EVPI as previously discussed. The EVPPI is essentially a measure of the sensitivity of the decision problem to the uncertainty in particular parameters. However, it has a number of advantages over other measures of sensitivity that are available. Firstly, it does not require or assume a linear relationship between the parameter and the model output (net-benefit). Indeed, by using the general approach outlined above, EVPPI can be established for any nonlinear or discontinuous relationship with net-benefit. Secondly, unlike other measures of sensitivity, the EVPPI is driven by decision uncertainty and the impact of parameter uncertainty on decisions. In this sense it combines both the notion of the importance of a parameter and the uncertainty surrounding its value. Finally, the approach generates estimates of the values of information which are consistent with the objectives of and the budget constraint on health care provision. Therefore, the value of information can be directly compared with the costs of conducting additional research. We have already shown how the EVPPI can start to indicate which research designs may be worth considering; however, establishing whether a particular type of research should be conducted requires an analysis of the value of sample information. This is introduced in Chapter 7.

6.4. **Identifying research priorities**

A number of methods for setting priorities in research and development of health care technologies have been proposed and some have been used to identify priority areas for research. These include measures of the burden of disease or the technology (Gross *et al.* 1999; Michaud *et al.* 2001); measures of the expected 'payback' from research (Buxton and Hannay 1997; Townsend *et al.* 1997; Davies *et al.* 2000); and estimates of the welfare losses due to variations in clinical practice (Phelps and Parente 1990). However, each of these proposed methods has serious methodological problems. Firstly, all of these proposed approaches view research simply as a means of changing clinical practice rather than considering research as providing additional information, which will reduce the uncertainty about what is appropriate clinical practice. Indeed, measures of 'payback' or welfare losses due to variations in clinical practice require the analysis to identify 'appropriate utilization' or which technology should be adopted a priori. These methods therefore implicitly assume that there is no uncertainty surrounding the decision that the proposed research is supposed to inform.

Secondly, these approaches, particularly measures of burden, attempt to identify research priorities using aggregate measures across broad clinical areas. However, the information generated by evaluative research is only valuable if it informs specific clinical decisions for specific groups of patients. Aggregate measures fail to recognize that the value of research in a clinical area is simply made up of the value of research about each of the constituent clinical decision problems faced within that area. Therefore, simply because aggregate measures such as burden of disease may suggest a clinical area is a 'high' priority, it does not mean that specific evaluative research relating to any one clinical decision problem will be valuable. Similarly, proposed research to inform a particular decision in a 'low' priority disease area may be very valuable.

In this sense, attempts to identify research priorities across broad clinical areas using aggregate indicators will be mistaken. What is required is a measure of the societal value of particular research, which can inform specific clinical decisions for defined groups of patients and value the additional information generated by research in a way, that is consistent with the objectives and the resource constraints of health care provision.

As we have seen in earlier sections of this chapter, the EVPI places an upper bound on the societal returns to additional evidence. These values are consistent with both the objective of the health care system and the budget constraint (represented by the cost-effectiveness threshold). Therefore, the value of information (the EVPI in this chapter and EVSI and ENBS in the next chapter) can be compared with the expected costs of further investigation. These estimates can be used to identify those areas of research and the type of research which will be most valuable and can inform the allocation of research and development resources within and between broad clinical areas. In addition, the value of information can be used to inform the allocation of resources between research and the provision of health care.

The use of value-of-information analysis has increased dramatically since 2000, particularly in health care (Yokota and Thompson 2004). Two recent pilot studies on the use of value-of-information analysis have been conducted in the UK to demonstrate the benefits and feasibility of using this type of approach to inform policy decision within the UK. The UK National Co-ordinating Centre for Health Technology Assessment (NCCHTA) which identifies research priorities and commissions research for the UK NHS, commissioned a pilot study on the use of decision analysis to inform its research prioritization process (Claxton *et al.* 2004). NICE also commissioned a pilot study of value-of-information analysis to support the institute's research recommendations made as part of its guidance to the NHS in England and Wales and to inform the deliberations of the NICE Research and Development Committee (Claxton *et al.* 2005*a*).

6.4.1. Recent policy experience

In many countries, decisions to adopt, reimburse or issue guidance on health technologies are increasingly based on explicit cost-effectiveness analysis using a decision analytic framework. A number of countries now request manufacturers of health care technologies to provide evidence on cost-effectiveness in support of applications for funding by the health care system. This approach was first used in Australia and Ontario for decisions about the funding of new medicines (CDHHCS 1992; Ontario Ministry of Health 1994). The approach has also been used by several managed care groups in the USA (Langley *et al.* 1999). All these agencies, including the Food and Drug Administration in the USA, consider whether the evidence used to support claims of cost-effectiveness is sufficient basis for the decision to reimburse, issue guidance or allow claims to be made (Claxton *et al.* 2005*b*). A prime example is the UK National Institute for Health and Clinical Excellence, where recent guidance on the methods of technology appraisal reflect the importance of representing decision problems explicitly, and of synthesizing evidence from a range of sources. One feature of the guidance is the development of 'reference case' requirements for analysis. The reference case in the NICE guidance includes decision analytic modelling, synthesis of evidence from various sources, and the characterization of uncertainty through probabilistic analysis. Although explicit valuation of additional evidence through value-of-information analysis is not required, it is recommended in order to inform the research recommendations that NICE issues alongside its guidance on technologies:

> Candidate topics for future research can be identified on the basis of evidence gaps identified by the systematic review and cost-effectiveness analysis. These may be best prioritized by considering the value of additional information in reducing the degree of decision uncertainty.

(NICE 2004)

In fact almost all the Technology Assessment Reports commissioned by NICE already include decision analysis and synthesis of evidence. A number have also included probabilistic analysis and value-of-information analysis. More recently, NICE commissioned a pilot study of value-of-information analysis to support the Institute's research recommendations made as part of its Guidance to the NHS in England and Wales and to inform the deliberations of the NICE Research and Development Committee (Claxton *et al.*, 2005*a*). The purpose was to establish the feasibility and requirements of using value-of-information analysis to consider the possible implementation of this framework within the NICE processes.

The pilot study consisted of a series of six case studies based on a re-analysis of recent Technology Assessment Reports completed for NICE. These included: screening for age-related macular degeneration (AMD); glycoprotein IIb/IIIa antagonists for acute coronary syndrome (GPAs); clopidogrel and dipyridamole in the secondary prevention of occlusive vascular events (CLO); neurominidase inhibitors for the treatment of influenza (NIs); liquid based cytology screening for cervical cancer (LBC); and beta interferon and glatiramer acetate in the management of multiple sclerosis (MS).

Value-of-information analysis was successfully implemented for each of the six case studies using the type of nonparametric methods described previously. For each case study, this allowed comparison of the potential benefits of further research (EVPI) with the costs of further investigation and an indication of whether further research may be required to support guidance on use of the technology issued by NICE. The EVPI associated with the groups of parameters indicated the type of evidence that would be most valuable and, therefore, the type of studies that should be recommended. The pilot study also enabled comparisons to be made across different technology assessments (decision problems) and was able to inform the prioritization of the range of research recommendations made by the Institute. This type of analysis also enables some comparison between the value of investing resources in research or other activities, such as the provision of health service. In this sense the application of the methods described in this and earlier chapters, for a body such as NICE, provides a unified and coherent framework for prioritization of both research and the use of health care technologies.

The results of the pilot study illustrated many of the issues discussed previously in this chapter. For example, the value of research differed substantially across the six technology appraisals and ranged from £2.8m (LBCs) to £865m (CLO). In some cases the analysis indicated that further research should not be regarded as a priority, for example, the EVPI surrounding LBC following evidence from a previous pilot study was low (£2.8m) and no further research was required. In other cases it indicated that additional research should be regarded as a priority, for example, the EVPI surrounding CLO for stroke patients was high (£865m). In other cases, the analysis refocuses the original research recommendations, such as in the AMD case study, although further research appears to be potentially worthwhile, it is additional evidence about quality of life with and without photodynamic therapy, rather than the performance of self-screening itself which is valuable.

The analysis also indicated which comparators should be included in future research and also suggested other parameters that could be excluded. For example, the value of information for NIs was significant (£66.7m) but it is further evidence about quality of life with influenza which is most important (£44.3m), rather than additional evidence about the effect on symptoms. Although there is some value in further randomized control trials (RCTs) on the effect of oselativir and amantadine on symptoms (£0.43m and £0.23m respectively), there is no value in further trials of zanamivir. Similarly in the MS case study, although there is value in additional RCT evidence of the effect on progression of the disease, it is the effect of copaxone and betaferon which should be regarded as a priority (£14m and £13.6m respectively). In this case, however, evidence about cost of care and relapse, and quality of life are also valuable. For these parameters, further research would not require experimental design and may be less costly to acquire (£10m and £6m respectively) so may be regarded as priorities.

Estimates of value of information for the decision problem and for groups of parameters were also presented for relevant patient subgroups, for example, the value of information differed across the patient groups considered in the CLO case study (from £856m to £240m). This suggests that further research on the stroke and myocardial infarction subgroups should be regarded as a priority, although research on the TIA and PAD subgroups may also be worthwhile. Similarly, the value of additional evidence for AMD differs by visual acuity (from £6.2m to £15.3m), and suggests that additional research should include those subgroups with lower starting visual acuity.

The analysis also indicates which endpoints should be included in further research. For example, in the GPA case study further research is valuable and should be regarded as a priority. It also indicated that it is RCT evidence of the effect of GPA as medical management and clopidogrel which is most valuable. However, it also indicates that the mortality endpoint for patients with non-acute PCI should be the primary endpoint in any future trial.

A number of case studies presented scenarios to explore alternative views of the relevant evidence. These included inclusion of related and 'unrelated events' in the assessment of CLO and impact of restricting consideration of evidence at 6 months in GPAs; different structural assumptions regarding the mechanism of action, such as the additive nature of information gains during screening for AMD; as well as the impact on value of information when relevant alternatives may have been excluded from the original scope of the appraisal, such as including the potential role of clopidigrel in the GPA case study. These examples demonstrated that even when this type of structural uncertainty has a limited impact on the estimates of cost-effectiveness, it can still have substantial impact on the value of information. This indicates the importance of accounting for structural uncertainty and, if possible, representing these issues as additional uncertain parameters within the model. The parameterization of structural uncertainty enables the analysis to address the question of the value of generating evidence that can resolve these uncertain assumptions (Carlin and Chib 1995).

A more detailed discussion of the results and the implications for research prioritization including the implications for the design of any future research in terms of features such as the relevant patient groups and comparators, and whether experimental design was likely to be required in each of the areas, can be found in full reports (Claxton *et al.* 2004, Claxton *et al.* 2005a). Both pilot studies also highlighted a number of methodological and computation challenges faced when applying value-of-information methods to policy-relevant decision problems in a timely way. However, it should be recognized that the key challenges for this type of analysis are not primarily the value-of-information methods themselves, but issues associated with structuring decision problems, synthesis of evidence and the characterization of uncertainty (required for estimating costs and effects as well as value of information).

Overall, the pilot studies demonstrated that the framework of decision analysis and value-of-information analysis can be applied to policy-relevant decisions in a timely way to provide results which can inform both the decision of whether a technology should be adopted based on existing evidence and whether more evidence is required to support that decision in the future. The studies also illustrate that the amount and type of evidence needed to inform decisions about health technologies is essentially an empirical question and different amounts and types of evidence will be needed for different technologies, applied to different patient groups in different circumstances.

6.4.2. **Necessary but not sufficient condition**

The EVPI discussed in this chapter and presented in these pilot studies only places an upper bound on the returns to further research. This provides a necessary condition for conducting further research where additional research about the decision problem as a whole or research about particular endpoints may be worthwhile if the EVPI or EVPPI exceeds the cost of conducting further research. However, to establish a sufficient condition: decide if further research will be worthwhile and identify efficient research design; we need to consider the marginal benefits and marginal cost of sample information.

The same framework of value-of-information analysis can be extended to establish the expected value of sample information for particular research designs and to compare these marginal benefits of research with the marginal costs (Claxton 1999; Ades *et al.* 2004). This type of analysis provides a societal payoff to alternative designs and can be used to establish optimal sample size, optimal allocation of patients within a clinical trial, appropriate follow-up and which endpoints should be included in the design. Indeed, this framework can be used to identify a portfolio of different types of studies, which may be required to provide evidence sufficient to support the use of a health care technology.

6.5. **Summary**

This chapter has argued that the conventional rules of inference are inappropriate for adopt/do not adopt decisions in health care decision making because of the potential opportunity costs associated with failing to implement cost-effectiveness decisions. As an alternative, it was argued that there are in fact two related, but distinct decisions: firstly, whether to adopt an intervention now, given the current state of knowledge concerning an intervention's cost-effectiveness; and secondly, whether additional information is required to support such adoption decisions in the future. The first type of decision (in the absence of serious concerns over reversibility) should be made on the basis of expected values in order to minimize opportunity costs. The second, requires consideration of the value of obtaining information and an upper bound on the returns to future research was established: the expected value of perfect information. This was argued to be a necessary condition for funding future research – in the next chapter we consider the sufficient condition for funding additional research.

6.6. **Exercise: calculating expected value of perfect information for the total hip replacement model**

6.6.1. **Objective**

The purpose of this exercise is to show how the model you have already developed can be adapted to calculate the expected value of perfect information (EVPI). As a first step, the overall EVPI for the model is calculated in order to summarise the overall importance of uncertainty for decision making. Secondly, the EVPI for individual parameters (or groups of parameters) can be calculated in order to examine the individual contribution of different parameter (combinations) to the overall uncertainty.

The step-by-step guide below will take you through the following stages for calculating expected value of information for the overall decision problem and for the parameters of the decision model:

1. Calculating per patient EVPI from simulation output.
2. Calculating the effective population and population EVPI.
3. Plotting EVPI as a function of the ceiling ratio.
4. EVPI for a parameter (EVPPI).
5. Plotting EVPPIs.

There are two templates for this exercise. Begin with the file *Exercise 6.6a – template.xls* for parts 1–3 above. Once complete, you will be prompted to open *Exercise 6.6b – template.xls* to continue the exercise.

6.6.2. **Step-by-step guide**

1. Calculating per patient EVPI from simulation output

In the template file you will find that we have returned to the model from Exercise 5.7 – where there is one new prosthesis to compare with the standard prosthesis. Move to the *<Simulation>* worksheet, which you should recognize from the previous exercise. Recall that, under a decision theoretic approach, it is the expected outcome that should guide the decision. That is, we will use the new prosthesis if it has an expected net-benefit that is greater than that of the standard prosthesis. However, due to uncertainty, sometimes we will make the wrong decision and the losses associated with the wrong decision are the net benefits forgone.

    i. In row 4 of the net-benefit columns (X to Z), record the mean net-benefit across the 1000 Monte Carlo simulations.

    ii. In the EVPI column (AK) calculate the maximum of the net benefits observed for standard or NP1 for each of the 1000 simulations (if we think of each simulation if like a 'realization of a state of the world' then this column represents net benefits under perfect information – where we always choose the prosthesis with the greatest net-benefit).

    iii. Now calculate the mean across the net benefits we would have under perfect information in cell AK4.

    iv. Finally, in cell AK1, calculate the difference between the mean of the maximized net benefits and the maximum of the mean values (X4 and Y4) – this gives the EVPI for the individual.

2. Calculating the effective population and population EVPI

Of course, there will be more than one patient eligible for a particular treatment. Therefore, the individual patient EVPI must be inflated by the effective population, which is a function of the eligible patients per annum and the expected lifetime of the technology. For the hip replacement example, we are going to assume an effective technology life of 10 years with 40 000 new patients eligible for treatment each year.

    i. In column AN link the cell showing the 40 000 patients per annum to the individual years of the technology lifetime and discount the population.

    ii. Sum the result in cell AN4 to give the effective population (discounted) over the lifetime of the technology.

    iii. Finally, multiply this effective population by the individual EVPI in cell AK1 to give the EVPI for the population in cell AP1.

3. Plotting EVPI as a function of the cost-effectiveness threshold

As EVPI is calculated using net-benefit and net-benefit is a function of the unknown cost-effectiveness threshold it is important to estimate EVPI as a function of the cost-effectiveness threshold.

    i. If you have calculated everything correctly so far, the population EVPI should automatically change when you enter a new value for the cost-effectiveness threshold in cell Z1. Test this, and when you are satisfied all is well, run the macro 'EVPI' which will use cost-effectiveness thresholds from column AP and record the corresponding EVPI in column AQ.

    ii. Now plot these results on the figure template *<EVPI>*.

   iii. Notice the peak in EVPI – where does this occur?

4. EVPI for a parameter (EVPPI)

The overall EVPI for the model is a useful upper limit on returns to future research. However, of crucial importance is which particular parameters (or groups of related parameters) are most important in terms of having the greatest value of information. EVPPI approaches are designed to look at just that. They work by looking at the value of information of the remaining parameters of the model if we assume perfect information for the parameter of interest.

  Begin by opening up the template file '*Exercise 6.6b – Template.xls*'. In this exercise, the approach is illustrated using the effectiveness parameter for the new prosthesis rrNP1. The exercise will get you to manually run through a looped exercise of obtaining estimates of net-benefit assuming that the value of rrNP1 is known. This may begin to appear repetitive – but the aim is to get a full appreciation of the approach before running a pre-written macro which will do the same thing but many more times (the aim is to get an understanding of the process rather than to give you practice in macro writing!)

     i. Start by checking the cost-effectiveness threshold value in cell Z1 is set to 2200 (this value is chosen to give a high EVPI for this part of the exercise).

    ii. We wish to estimate the effect of certain knowledge of rrNP1 on reducing the expected cost of uncertainty. However, we are uncertain as to the true value of rrNP1, therefore the first step is to draw a value at random from the distribution of rrNP1. Note that this can be done simply by copying the value in cell C27 of the *<Parameters>* worksheet and using the *Paste special: values* command to enter this value into cell B27.

   iii. The model now has a constant value for rrNP1 (drawn from its estimated distribution). Now run the MCsimulation macro to estimate the effect of the joint uncertainty in all the remaining parameters of the model.

   iv. Copy the mean net benefits for each prosthesis (cells X4:Y4) into the AS6:AT6 cells, remembering to use the *Paste special: values* command.

    v. Now repeat steps (ii) to (v) nine more times to give ten mean net benefits for different draws from the distribution of rrNP1. Record these values in AS7:AT15.
      Hint: if your PC is slow, such that this is taking a long period of time, reduce the number of times you do this looping before progressing to the next step.

vi. Now average across these ten evaluations of net-benefit to calculate the mean overall net-benefit over the draws from the distribution of rrNP1. Record these values in cells AS4:AT4. Note that these values are equivalent to the mean net benefits over all uncertainty in all parameters (as uncertainty over rrNP1 has been reintegrated).

vii. In cells AU6:AU15, find the maximum of the net benefits in columns AS and AT for the ten realizations you have obtained. This is the perfect information payoff given certainty over rrNP1. Calculate the mean value in cell AU4.

viii. The EVPPI for an individual patient is now calculated by subtracting the expected payoff with uncertainty over all parameters (the maximum of cells AS4 and AT4) from the expected payoff with perfect information about rrNP1 (cell AU4). Enter this formula in cell AX7 and multiply by the effective population (cell AN4) to give the EVPPI on rNP1 for the population.

ix. Copy this EVPPI from cell AX7 and paste into the EVPPI table (cell AX11) using the *Paste special: values* command.

x. The final step relates to 'tidying up' the model (this is crucial before moving on to the next section). Copy the formula from cell B26 on the parameters worksheet down to cell B27. This returns the rrNP1 from a deterministic draw to the deterministic mean or probabilistic value (depending on the value of the switch in cell D3).

5. Plotting EVPPIs

Now that you understand the process behind calculating EVPPIs, take a moment to examine the macros recorded for you in the spreadsheet by opening the visual basic editor. You will see a macro for six different parameters/ groups of parameters (where parameters are related, such as utilities or survival parameters, it makes sense to consider their EVPPIs together). An overall macro called 'partialEVPI' will run the full set of six EVPPI macros and record the results in the table AX11:AX16.

i. When you are happy with what the macros are doing, run the '*partialEVPI*' macro.

Note: this macro runs 100 Monte Carlo simulations by 100 draws from the parameter (group) of interest. It will therefore take a while to complete – you may need to leave your computer running for some time! However – and this is very important – accurate estimation of EVPPIs takes many more runs than this – we would recommend at least 1000 inner and 1000 outer loops. Time to buy a faster computer – or employ someone with specific programming skills (we recognize our code suggestions are not the fastest possible, but we are not Visual Basic experts!)

ii. When the macro has finished running, plot the results of the EVPPI analysis in the *<partialEVPI>* worksheet template as simple bar chart.

References

Ades, A. E., Lu, G. and Claxton, K. (2004) 'Expected value of sample information in medical decision modelling', *Medical Decision Making*, 24: 207–227.

Burles A., Clark W., Preston C., *et al.* (2000) *Is zanamivir effective for the treatment of influenza in adults* (supplement). London, National Institute for Clinical Excellence.

Buxton, M. and Hanney, S. (1997) 'Assessing payback from Department of Health Research and Development: Second report'. HERG Research Report 24. Uxbridge, Brunel University.

Carlin, B. P. and Chib, S. (1995) 'Bayesian model choice via Markov chain Monte Carlo methods', *Journal of the Royal Statistical Society. Series B*, 57(3): 473–484.

Claxton, K. (1999*a*) 'The irrelevance of inference: a decision making approach to the stochastic evaluation of health care technologies', *Journal of Health Economics*, 18: 342–64.

Claxton, K. (1999*b*) 'Bayesian approaches to the value of information: implications for the regulation of new health care technologies'. *Health Economics*, 8: 269–274.

Claxton, K. and Thompson, K. A. (2001) 'A dynamic programming approach to efficient clinical trial design. *Journal of Health Economics*', 20: 432–448.

Claxton, K. and Posnett, J. (1996) 'An economic approach to clinical trial design and research priority setting', *Health Economics*, 5: 513–524.

Claxton, K., Neuman, P. J., Araki, S. S. and Weinstein, M. C. (2001) 'The value of information: an application to a policy model of Alzheimer's disease', *International Journal of Technology Assessment in Health Care*, 17: 38–55.

Claxton, K., Sculpher, M. and Drummond, M. (2002) 'A rational framework for decision making by the National Institute for Clinical Excellence', *Lancet*, 360: 711–715.

Claxton, K., Ginnelly, L., Sculpher, M. J, Palmer S. and Philips, Z. (2004) 'A pilot study on the use of decision theory and value of information analysis as part of the NHS Health Technology Assessment programme', *Health Technology Assessment*, 8(31): 1–103.

Claxton, K., Eggington, S., Ginnelly, L., Griffin, S., McCabe, C., Philips, Z., Tappenden, P. and Wailoo, A. (2005*a*) 'A pilot study of using value of information analysis to support research recommendations for the National Institute for Clinical Excellence'. Centre for Health Economics, Research Paper No 4, University of York.

Claxton K., Cohen J. T. and Neumann P. J. (2005*b*) 'When is evidence sufficient?' *Health Affairs*, (24); 1: 93–101.

Commonwealth Department of Health, Housing and Community Services (CDHHCS) (1992) *Guidelines for the pharmaceutical industry on preparation of submissions to the Pharmaceutical Benefits Advisory Committee*. Canberra, AGPS.

Davies, L., Drummond, M. F. and Papanikolaou, P. (2000) 'Prioritizing investments in health technology assessment', *International Journal of Technology Assessment in Health Care*, 16: 73–91.

Felli, J. C. and Hazen, G. B. (1998) 'Sensitivity analysis and the expected value of perfect information'. *Medical Decision Making*, 18: 95–109.

Fenwick, E., Claxton, K. and Sculpher, M. (2001) 'Representing uncertainty: the role of cost-effectiveness acceptability curves'. *Health Economics*, 10: 779–89.

Ginnelly, L., Claxton, K., Sculpher, M. J. and Golder, S. (2005) 'Using value of information analysis to inform publicly funded research priorities'. *Applied Health Economics and Health Policy*, 4: 37–46.

Gross, C. P., Anderson, GF, NR P. (1999) 'The relation between funding by the National Institutes of Health and the burden of disease', *New England Journal of Medicine*, 340: 1881–1887.

Howard, R. A. (1966) 'Information value theory', *IEEE Transactions on Systems Science and Cybernetics*, SSC-2, 22–26.

Langley, P. C. (1999) 'Formulary submission guidelines for Blue Cross and Blue Shield of Colorado and Nevada. Structure, application and manufacturer responsibilities', *PharmacoEconomics*, 16: 211–224.

Michaud C. M., Murray CJ, BR. B (2001) 'Burden of disease – implications for future research'. *Journal of the American Medical Association*; 285.

Ministry of Health (1994) *Ontario guidelines for economic analysis of pharmaceutical products*. Ontario, Ministry of Health.

National Institute for Clinical Excellence (NICE) (2000) 'Guidance on the use of zanamivir (Relenza) in the treatment of influenza', *Technology Appraisals Guidance* 15. London, NICE.

National Institute for Clinical Excellence (NICE) (2004) *Guide to the methods of technology appraisal*. London: NICE.

O'Hagan, A. and Luce, B. (2003) *A primer on Bayesian statistics in health economics and outcomes research*. Bethesda, MD, MedTap International.

Phelps, C. E. and Parente, S. T. (1990) 'Priority setting in medical technology and medical practice assessment', *Medical Care*, 28: 703–723.

Pratt J., Raiffa, H. and Schlaifer, R. (1995) *Statistical decision theory*. Cambridge, MA, MIT Press.

Raiffa, H. and Schlaifer, R. (1959) *Probability and statistics for business decisions*. New York, McGraw-Hill.

Sculpher, M. J. and Claxton, K. (2005) 'Establishing the cost-effectiveness of new pharmaceuticals under conditions of uncertainty – when is there sufficient evidence?' *Value in Health*, 8: 433–446.

Thompson, K. M. and Evans, J. S. (1997) 'The value of improved national exposure information for perchloroethylene (perc): a case study for dry cleaners', *Risk Analysis*, 17: 253–271.

Thompson, K. M. and Graham, J. D. (1996) 'Going beyond the single number: using probabilistic risk assessment to improve risk management', *Human Ecology Risk Assessment*, 24: 1008–1034.

Townsend, J. and Buxton, M. (1997) 'Cost-effectiveness scenario analysis for a proposed trial of hormone replacement therapy', *Health Policy*, 39: 181–94.

Yokota, F. and Thompson, K. M. (2004) 'Value of information literature analysis: a review of applications in health risk management', *Medical Decision Making*, 24: 287–298.

Chapter 7

Efficient research design

In this chapter we establish a sufficient condition for deciding to conduct further research and identify efficient research design. To do so we need to consider the expected benefits and costs of sample information. The value of sample information and the expected net benefits of sampling are outlined in the following section. This section considers the case where incremental net-benefit is normally distributed, as well as the calculation of the expected value of sample information for parameters or groups of model parameters based on conjugacy assumptions. These methods are then applied to the simple model of zanamivir, which was introduced in Chapter 6. This example demonstrates how measures of the societal payoff from research can be used to identify efficient research designs. Additional issues for research design that can be addressed within the general framework offered by considering the value of sample information are discussed in the final section.

7.1. Expected value of sample information (EVSI)

In Chapter 6 we saw that the expected value of perfect information (EVPI) places an upper bound on the returns to further research. This provides a necessary condition for conducting further research, where additional research about the decision problem as a whole, or research about particular parameters or groups of parameters, may be worthwhile if the EVPI or expected value of perfect information for a parameter(s) (EVPPI) exceeds the cost of conducting further research. However, to establish a sufficient condition, decide if further research will be worthwhile and identify efficient research design we need to consider the marginal benefits and marginal costs of sample information.

The same framework of value-of-information analysis can be extended to establish the expected value of sample information for a sample of n (EVSI|n), for particular research designs. These expected benefits of research can be compared with the expected costs of sampling (Cs|n). The difference between the EVSI|n and Cs|n is the expected net-benefit of sampling for a sample size of n (ENBS|n). The ENBS|n can be regarded as the societal payoff to research and can be calculated for a range of samples, sizes and for alternative designs. It can be used to establish optimal sample size, optimal allocation of patients within a clinical trial, appropriate follow-up and which endpoints should be included in the design. Indeed, this framework can be used to identify a portfolio of different types of studies, which may be required to provide sufficient evidence to support the use of a health care technology. It is then possible to answer questions such as whether an additional clinical trial is required; and if so, should an economic evaluation be conducted alongside the new trial; and what is the optimal follow-up, sample size and allocation of entrants between the arms of the proposed trial?

7.1.1. **EVSI when net-benefit is normally distributed**

The expected benefit of sample information can be regarded as the resulting reduction in the cost of uncertainty surrounding the choice between alternatives j. For an individual patient, the expected benefits of a sample of n allocated between a new technology (alternative $j = 2$) and current practice, (alternative $j = 1$) in a proposed trial where $n_{(2)}$ are allocated to $j = 2$ and $n - n_{(2)}$ are allocated to $j = 1$, can be expressed as the expected value of sample information (EVSI$|n, n_{(2)}$). If incremental net-benefit is normally distributed then we can use analytic solutions similar to those described in Chapter 6 when we are considering samples of incremental net-benefit (Raiffa and Schlaifer 1959; Claxton and Posnett 1996; Claxton 1999):

$$\text{EVSI}|n, n_{(2)} = \lambda . \sqrt{(V|n, n_{(2)})\sigma 0} . L(D|n, n_{(2)}),$$

where:

λ = cost-effectiveness threshold

$$D|n, n_{(2)} = |\eta 0|/(\sigma 0 . \sqrt{(V|n, n_{(2)})}),$$

η_0 = prior mean incremental net health benefit

$$V|n, n_{(2)} = \sigma_0^2 / (\sigma_0^2 + (\sigma_{(2)}^2 / n_{(2)}) + \sigma_{(2)}^2 + (\sigma_{(1)}^2 / n - n_{(2)}))$$

σ_0^2 = prior variance of the incremental net-benefit (η_0).

The $\sigma_{(2)}^2$ and $\sigma_{(1)}^2$ are the population variances surrounding the net-benefit of alternative $j = 2$ and $j = 1$, respectively, so that as sample size increases $V|n, n_{(2)}$ tends to 1 and the expression for EVSI approaches the EVPI. In other words, perfect information can be regarded as an infinite sample and is the upper bound to EVSI.

As with EVPI, the expected value of sample information also has public good characteristics (it is nonrival), and can be used to inform the treatment decision of current and future patients who are not enrolled in this proposed trial. The value of sample information for the population of current and future patients over the effective lifetime of the technology (T) can be established based on estimates of the incidence of patients or episodes (I) in each period (t) discounted at rate r.

It should be noted that those patients who are enrolled in the trial in each period (n_t) will not be able to benefit from the information generated by the research because they will have already received treatment:

$$\text{Population EVSI}|n,\ n_{(2)} = \text{EVSI}|n,\ n_{(2)}.\Sigma_{(t\,=\,1,\,2,\,\ldots,\,T)}(I_t - n_t)/(1+r)^t.$$

Therefore, increasing the sample size provides more information for the population of patients (or episodes of illness) who are not enrolled in the trial, but it also 'uses up' those who would otherwise benefit from the sample information. The resource cost of a sample of n with $n_{(2)}$ allocated to $j = 2$ ($\text{Cs}|n$, $n_{(2)}$) includes the fixed costs of proposed research (Cf), the marginal (incremental) treatment costs compared with current clinical practice ($C_2 - C_1$) and marginal reporting costs (Cr):

$$\text{Cs}|n,\ n_{(2)} = \text{Cf} + (C_2 - C_1).n_{(2)} + \text{Cr}.n.$$

In this case the cost function is very simple with a fixed element and constant marginal costs. However, more complex cost functions can be easily incorporated. The societal payoff to proposed research or the expected net benefits of sampling ($\text{ENBS}|n$, $n_{(2)}$) is simply the difference between the expected benefits and expected cost of sampling:

$$\text{ENBS}|n,\ n_{(2)} = \text{EVSI}|n,\ n_{(2)} - \text{Cs}|n,\ n_{(2)}.$$

It is now possible to establish a sufficient condition for conducting further research and decide whether an additional study would be efficient. If the $\text{ENBS}|n$, $n_{(2)} > 0$ for any sample size and allocation of the sample between the arms of the trial, then further experimental research will be efficient. As well as providing a sufficient condition for deciding whether further evidence is required to support a decision to adopt a technology, this type of analysis also indicates what type of research is needed and how it should be designed. It provides a framework for the efficient design of clinical trials based on the societal payoff to research. In this case the optimal sample size (n^*) for this proposed research will be where ENBS reaches a maximum ($\text{ENBS}|n^*$, $n_{(2)}^*$), given that the trial entrants are allocated optimally ($n_{(2)}^*$) between the two arms of the trial. In fact, ENBS can be used to choose between alternative designs across a range of dimensions of research design including optimal follow-up; which endpoints should be included in the trial, when to stop a sequential trial; and, in principle, the optimal portfolio of different types of study, which can inform the decision problem. This discussion has outlined the conceptual issues and the use to which estimates of EVSI and ENBS can be put. However, in decision models it is very unlikely that net benefits will be normally distributed and it is more useful to focus on the value of acquiring sample information about groups of particular model parameters rather than directly on incremental net-benefit itself.

7.1.2. **EVSI for conjugate distributions**

For the same reasons as outlined in Chapter 6, net-benefit is very unlikely to be normally distributed and is unlikely to have a parametric distribution at all. The simple analytic framework outlined above is also based on sampling incremental net-benefit directly rather than sampling the uncertain parameters that determine net-benefit. In decision models, net-benefit is a function of many parameters and it is more useful to focus on the value of sample information associated with particular parameters or groups of model parameters. The approach outlined below is very similar to EVPPI and requires, for each proposed research design, the prediction of possible sample results, the possible posterior distributions which could result from these sample results and the associated net benefits (Pratt *et al.* 1995; Berry and Stangl 1996; Ades *et al.* 2004).

This approach to EVSI simply asks what the payoff (expected net-benefit) would be if we could base our decision on having additional sample information. We can do this by predicting the possible sample results we would get from a particular study with a sample size of *n*. We can combine our prior with each of these possible sample results to form a number of possible predicted posterior mean values (one for each predicted sample result) (Gelman *et al.* 1995; O'Hagan and Luce 2003). For each of these possible posteriors we can calculate the expected net-benefit of our decision. We do not know which of these predicted posteriors will result from the sample of *n* so we average the net benefits across them. The difference between the expected net benefits of our decision based on the predicted posteriors and the expected net benefits based on current information is the EVSI for a sample of *n* (Pratt *et al.* 1995; Ades *et al.* 2004).

More formally, suppose we were interested in the value of sample information about θ (initially imagine that θ is a single parameter and the only uncertain parameter in the model). A sample of *n* on θ will provide a sample result *D*. If we knew what the result of the sample would be in advance, then we could choose the alternative with the maximum expected net-benefit when these expected net benefits are averaged over the posterior distribution of the net-benefit of each treatment j given the sample result D:

$$\max_j E_{\theta|D} NB(j, \theta).$$

However, we do not know the actual results of the sample in advance (we do not know which value D will take). Therefore, the expected value of a decision taken with the sample information is found by averaging these maximum expected net benefits over the distribution of possible values of D; that is, the expectation over the predictive distribution of the sample results D conditional on θ, averaged over the prior distribution (possible values) of θ:

$$E_D \max_j E_{\theta|D} NB(j, \theta).$$

So the EVSI is simply the difference between the expected value of a decision made with sample information and the expected value with current information:

$$E_D \max_j E_{\theta|D} NB(j, \theta) - \max_j E_\theta NB(j, \theta).$$

However, models include more than one uncertain parameter and this approach can be extended to consider the value of sample information about a parameter or a subset of the parameters φ with remaining uncertain parameters in the model ψ. If φ and ψ are independent, then a sample of n on φ will provide a sample result D. If we knew D then expected net benefits are averaged over the prior distribution of ψ and the posterior distribution of φ given the sample result D:

$$\max_j E_{\psi, \varphi|D} NB(j, \varphi, \psi).$$

As we do not know which value D will take we must take the expectation of the maximum expected net benefits over the predictive distribution of D conditional on φ, averaged over the prior distribution of φ.

$$E_D \max_j E_{\psi, \varphi|D} NB(j, \varphi, \psi)$$

As before, the expected value of sample information is the difference between the expected value of a decision with sample information and the expected value of a decision based on current information:

$$E_D \max_j E_{\psi, \varphi|D} NB(j, \varphi, \psi) - \max_j E_\theta NB(j, \theta).$$

It should be clear from this discussion that EVSI requires predicted sample results to be combined with the prior information about a parameter to form predicted posteriors. For this reason we restrict discussion in this chapter to those situations where the likelihood for the data (in this case predicted sample results) is conjugate with the prior so there is an analytic solution to combining the prior with the predicted sample to form the predicted posterior (Gelman *et al.* 1995; O'Hagan and Luce 2003). If the prior and likelihood are not conjugate then there is no simple analytic solution and the computational burden of using numerical methods to form predicted posteriors is considerable (Ades *et al.* 2004).

Even with conjugacy EVSI still requires intensive computation. This is because in a similar way to EVPPI we have an inner and outer loop of expectation. However, EVSI is more intensive than EVPPI because we must first sample a value for D from the predictive distribution of D conditional on a value of φ, then sample from the prior distribution of ψ and the posterior distribution of φ given a sample result D (the inner loop). Then we must sample a new value for D from the predictive distribution of D conditional on a new value of φ and rerun the inner loop. This must be repeated until we have sampled sufficiently from the distribution (or joint distribution) of φ (the outer loop).

Of course, the EVSI described above is for a single study design and only one sample size. To establish the optimal sample size for a particular type of study, these calculations need to be repeated for a range of sample sizes to identify the point at which ENBS reaches a maximum. It should be noted that the EVPPI can provide an upper bound on the sample sizes that may be worth considering for particular groups of parameters. The EVPPI net of the fixed costs of research, divided by the marginal costs of sampling provides an upper bound on sample size. This is because the cost of sample sizes greater than this will exceed the EVPPI and the returns to any research study. Of course, if there are a number of different types of study which could generate information about different groups of parameters or studies with different follow-up periods or different allocations of sample between the alternatives, then these calculations would be needed for each possible design and for the range of possible sample sizes.

7.1.3. EVSI for linear models

The approach outlined above provides a general solution for nonlinear models given that the groups of parameters φ and ψ are (prior) independent (Ades *et al.* 2004). The computation for EVSI can be somewhat simplified if the model is either linear or multilinear in a similar way to EVPPI in Chapter 6.

If the model is linear and φ and ψ are independent, or if the model is multilinear and all the parameters (not just the subsets φ and ψ) are independent, then the inner loop can be simplified:

$$E_{\psi,\,\varphi|D}NB(j,\ \varphi,\psi)\ =\ NB(j,\ E(\varphi|D),\ E(\psi)).$$

In this case the net-benefit for a particular value of D can be calculated from the predicted posterior mean values of the parameters φ and the prior mean of the other parameters ψ. There is no need to sample from the predicted posterior distribution of φ or the prior distribution of ψ. A range of algorithms suitable for different levels of linearity in net-benefit is outlined in Ades *et al.* (2004).

7.2. **An example of EVSI**

The principles of using an analysis of EVSI can be illustrated using the simple example of zanamivir, which was discussed in Chapter 6. The National Institute for Clinical Excellence (NICE) considered zanamivir as a treatment for influenza in adults in 2000 and issued guidance (NICE 2000) imposing a number of restrictions and conditions on its use. In particular, treatment should only be offered when influenza is circulating in the community and for at-risk adults who present within 36 hours of the onset of influenza-like illness. At-risk adults were defined as those over the age of 65 or those with chronic respiratory disease, significant cardiovascular disease, immunocompromised and those with diabetes mellitus.

This guidance and the appraisal of zanamivir were based on the independent assessment report (Burles 2000). The assessment report identified nine randomized control trials but the evidence for at-risk adults is based on subgroup analysis of eight of the all-adult trials and one trial that only recruited adults with chronic respiratory disease. The trials reported time to alleviation of symptoms for the influenza-positive population, as well as the number of complications requiring antibiotics. The assessment report included fixed-effect meta-analysis for both these endpoints. None of the trials included effect on hospitalization, costs or quality of life. A simple decision tree model was presented in the assessment report where the proportion of influenza-positive patients (pip) presenting with influenza-like symptoms was based on a sponsored submission, the baseline risk of complication (pcs) and hospitalization (phs) was based on an observational data set. The reduction in complications requiring antibiotics was based on the log odds ratio from the fixed effect meta-analysis of the trials (LORc) and the same ratio was used to model reduction in hospitalizations (LORh). The reduction in symptom days (rds) for the influenza-positive population was based on a fixed effect meta-analysis, and the impact on quality of life of a symptom day (qsd) was based on an assumed impact on all dimensions of EQ5D. Resource use was based on published unit costs, hospital length of stay, and the number of GP visits.

This example was first introduced in Chapter 6 and the cost-effectiveness acceptability curve (CEAC) for this decision problem was illustrated in Fig. 6.1. The analysis of the population EVPI was illustrated in Fig. 6.3 and indicated that at a cost-effectiveness threshold of £50 000, further research may be potentially cost-effective. The analysis of the EVPIs for model parameters was illustrated in Figs 6.5 and 6.6 and suggested that further research about pip, phs, rds, upa and LORh may be worthwhile. In the following section we illustrate how the EVSI for sample information about each of these parameters can be calculated and illustrate the EVSI and ENBS for an additional clinical trial which would provide information on all parameters.

7.2.1. **EVSI for beta binomial**

The first uncertain parameter in this simple model is the probability that a patient is influenza-positive (pip). A beta distribution was assigned to this parameter in the probabilistic analysis. The analysis of the EVPPI in Chapter 6 indicated that additional information about this parameter may be worthwhile. Therefore, we could consider conducting an epidemiological study to estimate the probability of the patient being influenza-positive. To calculate the EVSI of such a study we must sample from the prior distribution:

$$\text{pip} \sim \text{Beta}(\alpha, \beta);$$

predict possible sample results (rip) using the binomial distribution:

$$\text{rip} \sim \text{Bin(pip, n)};$$

and then form predicted posterior distributions (pip'):

$$\text{pip}' \sim \text{Beta}((\alpha+\text{rip}), (\beta+\text{n}-\text{nrip})).$$

The pip' are the possible (predicted) posterior distributions for the probability of a patient being influenza-positive following the study with a sample size of n. With sample information we will be able to make a different decision for each predicted posterior pip'. Therefore, the expected value with sample information is found by calculating the expected net-benefit for a particular pip' and choosing the alternative with the maximum net-benefit. However, we do not know which of the possible posteriors will actually be the result of the research, so we must calculate the mean of these expected net benefits across all the values of pip'. The difference between the expected net benefits of our decision based on the predicted posteriors for pip (pip') and the expected net benefits based on current information is the EVSI for a sample of n.

In a nonmultilinear model the expected net benefits for a particular predicted posterior requires evaluation of net-benefit by sampling from the predicted posterior distribution. For a multilinear model (as in this case), however, the predicted posterior mean can be used to calculate the expected net benefits, substantially reducing the computation.

The relationship between the sample sizes considered, the prior and predicted posterior distribution and the EVSI are illustrated in Fig. 7.1 for the beta binomial case. Based on current information (the prior distribution) imagine that alternative j has the highest net-benefit. When a small sample size of $n = 1$ is considered, there are only two possible results from the binomial likelihood and the two possible posterior distributions will be similar to the prior distribution because the prior will dominate the limited sample information. It is, therefore, very unlikely that these possible posteriors will change the decision based on current information and thus EVSI will be low. In Fig. 7.1 we continue to choose alternative j irrespective of the results of the sample and EVSI = 0. However, when the sample size is larger ($n = 20$) there are a large number of possible sample results and the predicted posterior distributions can be some distance from the prior because the prior no longer

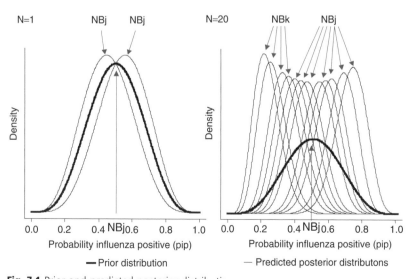

Fig. 7.1 Prior and predicted posterior distributions.

dominates the more substantial sample information. In this sense, as sample size increases we are more uncertain about where the posterior distribution might lie. It is now much more likely that the posterior will change the decision. In Fig. 7.1 some of the predicted posteriors change net-benefit so that we would choose alternative k rather than j. When we calculate the mean expected net-benefit over these predicted posteriors it will be higher than with current information. In other words, the EVSI will be positive and increases with n.

In fact, as sample size becomes very large, the predicted posterior can resolve anywhere across the prior distribution. The variance in the predicted posterior means approaches the prior variance and the EVSI for the parameter will approach the EVPPI – once again confirming our interpretation of EVPI and EVPPI.

The EVSI for an epidemiological study to estimate the probability that a patient is influenza-positive is illustrated in Fig. 7.2. This demonstrates that the EVSI will rise with sample size and approaches the EVPPI for pip as sample size becomes very large. Of course, the EVSI will also depend on the cost-effectiveness threshold and, just like the EVPPI, there is no clear monotonic relationship. For example, the EVSI will be lower at cost-effectiveness threshold of £40 000 and £60 000 reflecting the relationship between EVPPI and the cost-effectiveness threshold that was illustrated in Fig. 6.6.

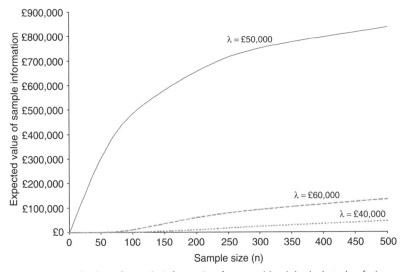

Fig. 7.2 Expected value of sample information for an epidemiological study of pip.

The probability of complication requiring hospitalization with standard care was also assigned a beta distribution and was associated with significant EVPPI in Fig. 6.6. The EVSI for an epidemiological study of the probability of hospitalization for patients with influenza can be calculated using the same approach, exploiting the conjugate relationship between the beta prior, the binomial likelihood and the predicted posterior beta distributions.

7.2.2. **EVSI for the normal distribution**

There is also uncertainty in the effectiveness of zanamivir and a normal distribution was assigned to the reduction in symptom days (rsd) for patients who are influenza-positive based on the results of a fixed effect meta-analysis of the clinical trials. The EVPPI associated with rsd in Fig. 6.6 suggested that further research may be worthwhile. We can use the same approach to consider the value of conducting a further clinical trial to provide a more precise estimate of rsd. To calculate the EVSI for a trial of n patients who are allocated equally between zanamivir and standard care, we must first sample from the prior distribution of rsd:

$$\text{rsd} \sim N(\mu_0, \sigma_0^2).$$

For each sample from this prior distribution we must predict possible sample results (μ_S) which will be normally distributed:

$$\mu_S \sim N(\text{rsd}, \sigma^2/n).$$

Then combine the prior with the predicted sample results to form a predicted posterior distribution which will also be normally distributed:

$$\text{rsd'} \sim N(\mu', I'),$$

where:

$$\mu' = ((\mu_0.I_0 + \mu_S.I_S)/(I_0 + I_S))$$
$$I_0 = 1/\sigma_0^2$$
$$I_s = 1/(\sigma^2/n)$$
$$I' = (n+m)/\sigma^2$$
$$m = \sigma^2.I_0.$$

As with pip, the EVSI for rsd is simply the difference between the expected net benefits of decisions based on the predicted posteriors for rsd and the expected net benefits based on current information.

The quality of life associated with influenza symptoms was also normally distributed and was also associated with significant EVPPI in Fig. 6.6. The EVSI for a study of quality of life in influenza-positive patients can be calculated using the same approach, exploiting the conjugate relationship between the prior, the likelihood and the predicted posterior distributions.

7.2.3. EVSI for log odds ratios

The effect of zanamivir on complications requiring hospitalization was associated with significant EVPPI in Fig. 6.6, which suggests additional research on this endpoint may also be worthwhile. A combination of the normal distribution and the beta binomial relationship enables the calculation EVSI for a clinical trial of n patients, which would estimate the log odds ratio of hospitalization for those treated with zanamivir compared with standard care. As the baseline probability, phs, has a beta prior and binomial likelihood and the LORh has a normal prior and normal likelihood, we can simply exploit the same principles outlined above: (i) sample from the beta prior on phs and the normal prior on LORh; (ii) calculate the prior on phz based on the sampled prior values of phs and LORh; (iii) use these sampled prior values of phz and phs to predict the results of the study from their respective binomial likelihood; (iv) use these results to calculate the predicted sample LORh; (v) combine the prior LORh with the predicted sample LORh to form a predicted posterior LORh; (vi) propagate the predicted posterior LORh through the model to calculate the expected net-benefit for this particular posterior; (vii) repeat this process to sample across the range of possible posteriors recording the expected net benefits from each; (viii) calculate the mean across these expected net benefits with the sample information. It should be noted that it is not possible to simply use the mean posterior LORh to calculate phz and therefore net-benefit in the model as this relationship is not linear. Therefore, either each predicted posterior distribution (not just the mean) must be propagated through the model or mathematical approximations (Taylor series expansion) can be used. More detail about EVSI for common data structures and mathematical approximations can be found in (Ades *et al.* 2004).

7.2.4. EVSI and research design

The EVSI for each of the parameters associated with a significant EVPPI in Chapter 6 and for which further research may be worthwhile are illustrated in Fig. 7.3. This demonstrates that the EVSI increases with sample size and approaches the EVPPI as sample size increases. Therefore, the EVSI will differ in the same way that EVPPI differed across model parameters when sample size is very large. However, at lower sample sizes this is not necessarily the case.

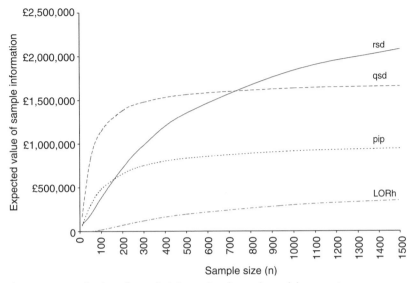

Fig. 7.3 Expected value of sample information for each model parameter.

In Fig. 7.3 when $n = 100$ the EVSI associated with rsd is lower than for pip or upa. This reflects that fact that there is already substantial prior information about rsd and that a further clinical trial with a small sample size is unlikely to change the decision and generate net-benefit (see Fig. 6.1). The pip and upa parameters are more uncertain, so that relatively small amounts of sample information can have a substantial effect on their posterior distribution and are more likely to have an impact on the decision and on expected net-benefit.

The methods we have just outlined mean that we can now think about designing research in an efficient way, taking account of the benefits and costs of different research designs. Indeed, we can calculate the EVSI for any parameter that is conjugate and consider the expected net benefits of sampling for studies that will inform individual parameters, for example, a epidemiological study for pip, a survey of quality of life for upa and a clinical trial to estimate rsd and LORh. However, many types of study will provide information about more than one parameter. For example, a clinical trial may include the rsd endpoint, but with sufficient sample size and follow-up could also estimate the log odds of complications requiring hospitalization.

The EVSI for a clinical trial that includes all the model parameters as endpoints is illustrated in Fig. 7.4. The EVSI when updating groups of parameters together is not simply the sum of the EVSI for the individual parameters (for the same reasons that the EVPPI for parameters will not sum to the decision EVPI).

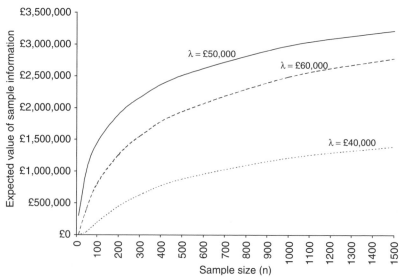

Fig. 7.4 Expected value of sample information for the decision problem.

But rather the difference between the expected net benefits of decisions based on the predicted posteriors for all the parameters and the expected net benefits based on current information. For this design, which provides information on all the uncertain parameters, the EVSI will approach the decision EVPI as sample size increases, confirming the interpretation that the perfect information is the upper limit on the value of sample information. Again, the relationship between EVSI and the cost-effectiveness threshold reflects the relationship illustrated in Fig. 6.3 for EVPI and demonstrates that a higher monetary valuation of health outcome does not necessarily mean a higher valuation of sample information.

So far this example has been used to illustrate how to estimate the benefit of sample information. However, by comparing the EVSI with the costs of sampling, we can identify optimal sample size where the ENBS reaches a maximum. This is illustrated in Fig. 7.5 for a clinical trial that includes all the parameters as endpoints, where the trial entrants are allocated equally between zanamivir and standard care (for a cost-effectiveness threshold of £50 000). The EVSI increases with sample size but ultimately at a declining rate. In this example the marginal costs of sampling with equal allocation are constant and the ENBS reaches a maximum of £2.4m at an optimal sample size of 1100. The fixed costs of the trial have been excluded as they will not change the optimal sample size. If the ENBS of £2.4m is greater than the fixed costs of this

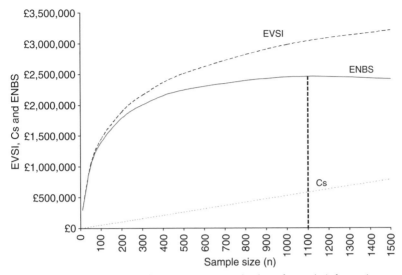

Fig. 7.5 Expected net-benefit of sampling, expected value of sample information, expected costs of sampling and optimal sample size.

research then the proposed trial can be can be considered cost-effective. We have met the sufficient condition for conducting further research.

As EVSI depends on the cost-effectiveness threshold, we would expect different ENBS and different optimal sample sizes for different thresholds. This is demonstrated in Fig. 7.6, which illustrates the ENBS and optimal samples size for three cost-effectiveness thresholds. Clearly the ENBS reflects the same type of relationship to the cost-effectiveness threshold as the EVPI in Fig. 6.3 and EVSI in Fig. 7.4. It shows that the value of research and the optimal sample size depends crucially on the cost-effectiveness threshold. It demonstrates that economic arguments are central to fundamental design decisions. In this example, despite the fact that the ENBS is lower for a threshold of £60 000 compared with £50 000 the optimal sample size increases. In general, however, there is no reason why there should be a monotonic relationship between the threshold and optimal sample size.

In this example we have only explored a small number of the possible research designs. So, although the ENBS at the optimal sample size in Fig. 7.5 is positive, indicating that this particular research design would be cost-effective and that further research is needed, it does not indicate whether there are other possible research designs that are more efficient (with higher ENBS). In fact, there are a large number of possible research designs, including different endpoints included in a clinical trial, alternative allocation of trial entrants

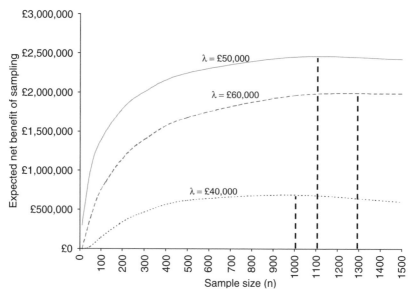

Fig. 7.6 Expected net-benefit of sampling and optimal sample size.

between the arms of the trial or a portfolio of different research designs addressing different uncertain model parameters. In principle, we could use this framework to choose the design that maximizes ENBS over all the dimensions of design space. These issues are discussed in the next section along with some of the computational challenges involved.

7.3. Design decisions

The concepts of EVSI and ENBS enable us to address some important research design issues, as well as providing a framework for considering the opportunity cost of ethical concerns about proposed research. This contrasts sharply with the more traditional approach to research design based on the power calculation. The effect size, which must be specified in the traditional power calculation, is not the effect that is expected, but what you wish to detect. However, there are no resource or opportunity costs of sampling specified. If asked what you wish to detect but at no cost, the only honest answer must be you wish to detect anything, however small. But as effect size approaches zero, the sample size required becomes unbounded. In practice, therefore, positive effect sizes are chosen in an essentially arbitrary way to achieve finite and 'manageable' sample sizes. In this sense, the traditional power calculation leads to only two sample sizes: infinite ones and arbitrary ones. In fact, most researchers with experience of using the tradition power calculation know how it is used in practice: (i) estimate potential grant funding for the project, take away the fixed costs and divide by marginal cost to find the sample size you can afford, and/or estimate the patients you will be able to recruit; (ii) solve for the effect size which can be detected at 5 per cent significance and 80 per cent power. In this sense, the traditional power calculation is bankrupt and dishonest (Claxton and Posnett 1996).

7.3.1. Fixed sample design

Previously we demonstrated that the optimal sample size will be where the ENBS reaches a maximum. This was illustrated in Fig. 7.4 for a clinical trial which included all the parameters in the simple decision model of zanamivir. However, the estimates of EVSI and ENBS were based on an equal allocation of the sample (trial entrants) between the two arms of this proposed trial (zanamivir and standard care). An equal allocation of sample between the arms of a proposed trial would be efficient if the marginal benefits and the marginal costs of allocating are the same across the arms of the trial. If the benefits and costs of allocation to the alternative arms differ then equal allocation will not be optimal.

The equal allocation of patients between experimental and control arms of a trial is often used and is implicitly justified by assuming that the variance of the outcome of interest for the control arm of the trial is the same as the experimental arm, so that the marginal benefits (reduction in sample variance) of assigning an additional trial entrant to either arm of the trial will be the same. However, there is little justification for this rule of precedent and there is no reason why the marginal costs and benefits of sampling should be the same across the arms of the proposed trial. For example, the costs of allocating trial entrants to the zanamivir arm will be higher due to the positive incremental costs of this technology. In addition, different parameters will be relevant to the zanamivir (e.g. RSD, LORc and LORh) and the standard care arms of the trial, so there is no reason to believe that the marginal benefits of allocating trial entrants will be the same either. Estimates of ENBS are therefore required for the range of possible allocations of each sample size considered. The optimal allocation will be the one that maximizes ENBS. Optimal allocation needs to be established for each sample size so that the optimal sample size, given that it will be allocated optimally between the arms of the trial, can be identified. In other words, we can use ENBS to identify the efficient design over these two dimensions of design space (optimal allocation and sample size) (Claxton 1999; Claxton and Thompson 2001). It should be recognized that optimal allocation of a given sample will depend on the cost-effectiveness threshold, as this will determine the weight placed on differences in the marginal costs and marginal benefits of allocating trial entrants to the arms of the proposed trial, demonstrating once again that fundamental design issues cannot be separated from economic concerns.

7.3.2. Sequential design

So far we have only considered a fixed sample design where the results of the trial are available at the end of the study after all entrants have been allocated and the sample size has been determined. There is a body of literature that considers the optimal allocation of trial entrants in sequential clinical trials where the results of the trial accumulate over time and can be used to assign entrants to the different arms (Armitage 1985). An example of this type of approach is Bather's 'play the winner rule' where patients are assigned to the arm of the trial which appears to be most effective given the accumulated trial results (Bather 1981). This approach, as well as others addressing the same problem and more recent dynamic programming approaches to this problem (Carlin *et al.* 1994), do not explicitly consider the marginal cost and benefits of sampling, and tend to focus on minimizing the potential health cost to individuals enrolled in the trial.

However, the framework of value-of-information analysis can also be usefully applied to sequential trial designs to establish the optimal allocation of each patient or group of patients and when to stop the trial. In principle an EVSI and ENBS calculation can be conducted after each result: the parameters are updated and the EVSI and ENBS are recalculated based on the new posterior distributions. The next patient or group of patients should simply be allocated to the arm that provides the highest ENBS. Patients should continue to be recruited and allocated in this way until the ENBS for the next patient or group of patients is zero. At this point it is no longer efficient to continue the trial. The trial should be then be stopped and the accumulated sample size and allocation will be optimal. In principle, this seems very straightforward and in many circumstances could lead to an optimal solution. However, it should be recognized that in deciding how to allocate the next patient, or whether to stop the trial, the EVSI calculation should take account of all the ways that the future trial entrants could be allocated as well. This is computationally very demanding and may require dynamic programming (Bellman *et al.* 1962; Claxton and Thompson 2001).

7.3.3. Data monitoring and ethics

Even when trials are not designed to be sequential there is often an opportunity to monitor the accumulated results for safety and to identify whether the trial should be stopped early on ethical grounds because one of the interventions has been demonstrated to be more effective. As should be clear from the previous discussion, the question of when to stop a trial can be addressed by calculating the ENBS given the accumulated evidence. If the ENBS is positive then it is efficient to continue the trial; if it is negative then the trial should be stopped.

Much of data monitoring and questions about the ethics of randomized trials are concerned with the implications for those individuals enrolled in the trial. However, the EVSI and ENBS calculations outlined above are primarily concerned with the benefits of information to the population of current and future patients. These approaches do not explicitly model the expected costs and benefits to individual trial entrants. It is possible to model the costs and benefits of those enrolled in the trial, but this issue of 'individual ethical concerns' may be more appropriately left for those who are responsible for the ethical approval. This approach, however, will allow us to establish the opportunity cost to 'collective ethics' of holding particular ethical concerns for trial entrants. For example, the ENBS of a proposed trial represents the opportunity cost to other current and future patients of failing to approve it on ethical grounds. Similarly the ENBS following data monitoring represents the opportunity cost of failing to continue the trial due to concerns for those enrolled.

7.3.4. Relevant alternatives

The framework offered by value-of-information analysis can also be used to identify which alternatives should be compared in a proposed clinical trial. The example of zanamivir conveniently considered only two alternatives. In most decision problems, however, there are potentially many possible strategies. Clearly, any economic evaluation should compare all relevant alternatives. However, it is not often made clear what does and what does not constitute a relevant alternative. In practice, many feasible alternatives are ruled out as irrelevant during the design of prospective research. If the identification of 'relevant alternatives' to be included in prospective research is either arbitrary, or uses implicit decision rules which are inconsistent with those that will be applied when the study is complete, then there is a danger that research will revolve around an arbitrarily selected subset of strategies. There is a real possibility that the optimal strategy may have already been ruled out of the analysis prematurely as an 'irrelevant alternative'. The evaluation of a particular clinical decision problem should, at least initially, consider all feasible alternatives, rather than focus only on those currently used or those identified as of interest in some arbitrary way. The 'relevant alternatives' that should be compared in prospective research should be identified explicitly and consistently.

If alternatives cannot be ruled out a priori but the prospective evaluation of all feasible alternatives is not possible or efficient, then this poses the question of which of the many competing alternative strategies should be considered 'relevant' and be compared in future research. We have already illustrated the use of EVPI in identifying a strategy which is not relevant and can be excluded in Table 6.2. However, most strategies will contribute to the EVPI and we will not be able to exclude them on these grounds. Optimal sample allocation based on ENBS enables relevant alternatives that should be compared in prospective research to be identified explicitly and consistently. Relevant alternatives can be defined as those where it will be efficient to allocate some of the sample in a subsequent evaluative trial. When it is not efficient to allocate patients to an arm of a trial, then that alternative can be safely ruled out as irrelevant (Claxton and Thompson 2001).

It is also worth noting the flaw in the notion that dominated programmes (whether strongly or extendedly dominated) can be excluded from an analysis and from subsequent research. It is possible that a dominated alternative will be relevant in subsequent evaluation (i.e. may have a high probability of being cost-effective), while a nondominated but not optimal alternative may not (i.e. may have a very low probability of being cost-effective). In these circumstances, the concept of dominance is not only unnecessary when using net-benefit, it is also potentially misleading. It is only by explicitly considering the marginal costs and benefits of sample information that a consistent and rational definition of what constitutes the set of relevant and irrelevant alternatives is available (Claxton and Thompson 2001).

7.3.5. **A portfolio of research designs**

The earlier discussion of EVSI and ENBS considered a single trial, which would provide sample information on all parameters in the decision model. However, this is only one possible design. The EVSI and ENBS could be considered for a trial that only included clinical endpoints such as rsd and LORc and LORh, which are particularly vulnerable to selection bias. In addition, rather than establish EVSI and ENBS for a clinical trial, we could consider a simple epidemiological study which would provide information about pip or a survey of quality of life with influenza to provide additional information about qsd. The ENBS and optimal sample size for these three additional potential study designs are illustrated in Fig. 7.7.

The ENBS and optimal sample size differ across these alternative studies. If we were restricted to choosing only one of the four possible study designs

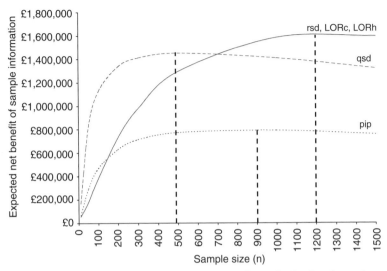

Fig. 7.7 Expected net-benefit of sampling and optimal sample size for alternative types of study.

we should choose the study with the highest ENBS. In this case, this would be the clinical trial that provided information on all parameters illustrated in Fig. 7.6. However, we could consider conducting a number of different studies to inform different parameters, specifically, a clinical trial to inform rsd, LORc and LORh, *and* an epidemiological study to inform pip *and* a survey to inform upa. It should be recognized that the ENBS for this portfolio of studies will not be the simple addition of the ENBS for each separate study in Fig. 7.7. Assuming that these three studies will report at the same time, so that the results of one cannot inform the results of the others, the ENBS would need to be calculated for each combination of sample sizes across the three studies. The optimal portfolio of research would be the combination of sample sizes across the studies that maximized ENBS. This clearly requires substantial computation, particularly if we also consider the optimal allocation of samples within, as well as between, studies.

A more realistic situation, however, is that the results of one study will be available before the other studies are completed. Indeed, it may be worth waiting until one study reports before initiating an other. In other words, as well as considering the optimal combination of studies, we can also consider the optimal sequence of studies within this portfolio. Now the computation is very demanding, as the EVSI for the first study depends on all the possible future studies that could be conducted given all the possible results of the first.

It should be clear from this discussion that although ENBS provides a powerful tool to identify optimal research design, the dimensions of this design space make this a computationally challenging task.

7.3.6. Development decisions

The discussion around value of information has been restricted to evaluative research and we have not explicitly considered the role of value of information in informing development decisions. In principle, value-of-information analysis can be used to inform the whole lifecycle of the development, evaluation and implementation of a health technology. Of course there will be substantial uncertainty surrounding the expected costs and effects of a technology which is in development. Therefore, a decision to continue to invest in developing a technology should be based not only on the expected payoff (expected net-benefit from a societal perspective) but also the value of information. For example, even if the expected payoff from a technology in development is negative, if the value of information is high then it may still be worthwhile conducting further research, as there is a chance that the technology will turn out to be cost-effective. The development of a technology should stop if the expected payoff is negative and the costs of further investigation exceed the value of information (i.e. it does not appear that it will be cost-effective and further research is unlikely to change this conclusion). In this way the framework of value-of-information analysis can be used to focus on those technologies which are likely to be worth developing and identify the type of research that is needed within the development programme.

Throughout Chapters 6 and 7, the value of information has been considered from a societal perspective, that is, based on maximizing net-benefit or equivalently maximizing health outcome subject to a resource constraint. However, there is no reason why the same type of analysis cannot incorporate other objectives, such as a commercial objective to maximize profit. For example, a commercial payoff function could be based on the licensing decision, modelled as a frequentist hypothesis test of efficacy; a reimbursement decision, based on expected cost-effectiveness; and sales (conditional on successful licensing and reimbursement), also a function of either expected effectiveness or cost-effectiveness. Once a commercial payoff function has been specified, the value-of-information calculations will provide the value of conducting further research from this commercial perspective. This can inform stop–go decisions at Phase II, the design of a portfolio of research which may be needed to support this decision and support licensing and reimbursement at Phase III.

As value of information can be estimated based on both commercial and societal payoffs to drug development decisions for a range of licensing and reimbursement rules, it can also be used to explore the type of regulatory regimens that will generate the socially optimal level of evidence to support a technology (Hawkins and Claxton 2003).

7.4. **Summary**

The purpose of this chapter has been to demonstrate how we can move from the necessary condition that the expected value of perfect information exceeds the cost of research to the sufficient condition that the marginal benefits of sampling exceed the marginal costs. The way in which the expected value of sample information can be calculated was then reviewed, drawing parallels with the calculation of the expected value of perfect information from the previous chapter. Examples of how to undertake these calculations were then given for different types of parameter distribution. Finally, it was demonstrated how the framework offered by the expected value of sample information approach could be brought to bear on a number of different design questions that naturally arise in health care evaluation research.

References

Ades, A. E., Lu, G. and Claxton, K. (2004) 'Expected value of sample information in medical decision modelling'. *Medical Decision Making*, 24: 207–227.

Armitage, P. (1985) 'The search for optimality in clinical trials'. *International Statistical Review*, 53:15–24.

Bather, J. A. (1981) 'Randomised allocation of treatments in sequential experiments', *Journal of the Royal Statistical Society B*, 43: 265–292.

Bellman, R. E. and Dreyfus, S. E. (1962) *Applied dynamic programming*, Princeton University Press.

Berry, D. A. and Stangl D. K. (1996) *Bayesian biostatistics*. New York: Marcel Dekker.

Burles A., Clark W., Preston C., *et al.* (2000) *Is zanamivir effective for the treatment of influenza in adults* (supplement). London, National Institute for Clinical Excellence.

Carlin, B.P., Kadane, J. B., and Gelfand, A. E. (1992) 'Approaches for optimal sequential decision analysis in clinical trials', *Biometrics*, 54: 964–975.

Claxton, K. (1999) 'The irrelevance of inference: a decision making approach to the stochastic evaluation of health care technologies', *Journal of Health Economics*, 18: 342–364.

Claxton, K. and Posnett, J. (1996) 'An economic approach to clinical trial design and research priority setting', *Health Economics*, 5, 513–524.

Claxton, K. and Thompson, K. A. (2001) 'A dynamic programming approach to efficient clinical trial design', *Journal of Health Economics*, 20, 432–448.

Gelman, A., Carlin, J. B., Stern, H. S. and Rubin, D. B. (1995) *Bayesian data analysis*. London, Chapman and Hall.

Hawkins, N. and Claxton, K. (2003) 'Optimal drug development programmes and efficient licensing and reimbursement rules: the role of value-of-information analysis', *Medical Decision Making*, 23(6): 564.

National Institute for Clinical Excellence (NICE) (2000) 'Guidance on the use of zanamivir (Relenza) in the treatment of influenza', *Technology Appraisals Guidance* No 15. London, NICE.

O'Hagan, A. and Luce, B. (2003) *A primer on Bayesian statistics in health economics and outcomes research*. Bethesda, MD, MedTap International.

Pratt, J., Raiffa, H. and Schlaifer, R. (1995) *Statistical decision theory*. Cambridge, MA, MIT Press.

Raiffa, H. and Schlaifer, R. (1959) *Probability and statistics for business decisions*. New York, McGraw-Hill.

Chapter 8

Future challenges for cost-effectiveness modelling of health care interventions

This book has attempted to introduce the reader to some of the more sophisticated aspects of applying cost-effectiveness models to health care decision problems relating to the implementation of new technologies. We started by briefly reviewing the common types of decision model employed for this task in Chapter 2 and went on to consider more sophisticated extensions to the standard 'cohort' model in Chapter 3. Chapter 4 considered how parameter uncertainty could be captured in our decision models through the use of parametric distributions, while Chapter 5 showed how this uncertainty in the input parameters of the model could be analysed in terms of the uncertainty relating to decision itself, principally through the use of CEACs. Chapter 6 argued that traditional rules of inference or consideration of Bayesian posterior probabilities have no role for decision making and that current adoption decisions should be made on the basis of expected values with additional research collected to support those decisions where it can be demonstrated that such additional information is valuable. Chapter 7 extended the value-of-information framework to consider the value of sample information and show that this framework has the potential to answer not only the question of whether additional information should be collected, but also the appropriate study design for doing so.

While the intention in writing this book was never to take a direct philosophical stand on the issue of statistical analysis of data, it should be clear to the reader that the methods and techniques we describe sit most comfortably in a Bayesian framework, with parameters assigned distributions to reflect their uncertainty, inferential decision rules abandoned and direct consideration given to the probability of error together with the consequences of error. Nevertheless, the typical reader we anticipated as the audience for this book was probably schooled (like us) in classical statistics, and could (like some of us) be working within departments dominated by the notions of 'evidence-based' medicine where confidence intervals and significance tests reign supreme.

Furthermore, the normative idea of 'evidence-based' medicine is one that we would sign up to in that our task in developing probabilistic cost-effectiveness models of health care interventions is to accurately describe the current evidence that bears on a particular decision problem rather than to include our own subjective priors, or those of our clinical colleagues. In the absence of hard data relating to a parameter, we feel most comfortable assigning a non-informative prior reflecting the absence of evidence. This recognizes that the analysts/decision makers are acting not for themselves, but on behalf of society as a whole. Perhaps our particular stance of adopting an informal approach to Bayesian methods may infuriate the purists, but our hope is that this will encourage more, rather than fewer, analysts to consider the merits that a Bayesian approach brings to the problem of health care evaluation.

In trying to bring together a text on cost-effectiveness modelling, representation of uncertainty and value-of-information analysis that is essentially practical in nature, there is an inherent danger that we give the impression that all the problems and issues are resolved. In truth, this is far from the case and our intention in this final chapter is to reflect on the challenges that are likely to face analysts attempting to implement the techniques we describe and the likely areas of future development. Below we consider future challenges under three broad headings: structuring of decision problems; evidence synthesis and uncertainty; and value-of-information techniques themselves.

8.1. **Structuring decision problems**

Identifying an appropriate structure for a decision problem is, of course, crucially important for estimating cost-effectiveness. A single structure for a model does not, exist, however, and different ways of structuring a model can have important consequences for the characterization of uncertainty and the subsequent value-of-information calculations. Indeed, the value of information will in general be highly sensitive to model specification, and a number of particular issues have been highlighted in recent applications of value of information.

Ensuring a sufficiently wide scope for the assessment to include all the relevant alternative strategies is particularly important. This includes other technologies as well as different clinical policies (e.g. start and stop criteria) for a single technology. As discussed in the previous two chapters, the exclusion of alternative strategies may not change the overall guidance on use of a technology, but in some cases it may have a substantial impact on the value of information and on any research recommendations.

Exploring and reflecting the additional uncertainty surrounding alternative but credible structural assumptions is also required. Even when the alternative assumptions may have limited impact on estimates of cost-effectiveness, they may have a more substantial impact on the value of information. This suggests that uncertainty, and therefore evidence, about the structural relationship may be as valuable as evidence about the model parameters. These types of uncertainty may be modelled as scenarios, or more usefully by assigning additional uncertain parameters to represent alternative assumptions. For example, in Chapter 3, the use of standard survival analysis methods for calculating Markov transition probabilities was introduced. Where there is uncertainty over the choice of functional form, then alternative functional forms could be included as scenarios in the model. Alternatively, a general form such as the Weibull function could be specified, and uncertainty over the functional form could be represented through the ancillary parameter. This approach enables this source of uncertainty to be fully integrated so that the value of information associated with these uncertainties can be established (Ginnelly and Claxton 2005). Nevertheless, such an approach raises the issues associated with the general problem of Bayesian model averaging (Draper 1995), in particular the issues associated with an infinite number of potential model structures.

Clearly, more complex model structures and computational expensive models make the characterization of uncertainty and value-of-information analysis more computationally demanding. As mentioned in Chapter 3, a number of approaches can be taken to overcome the computational problems, including the use of more efficient programming platforms, mathematical approximations and the use of emulators (Stevenson *et al.* 2004; O'Hagan *et al.* 2005). This raises the issue whether it is more appropriate to specify a highly complex model structure, such that some form of approximation is necessary to undertake the uncertainty and value-of-information analysis, or whether it is justifiable to use simplifying assumptions to keep the model manageable.

8.2. **Evidence synthesis and characterizing uncertainty**

Chapter 4 focused on fitting distributions to represent uncertainty in different types of parameters. Most of the simplified examples focused on fitting parameter distributions based on single data sources guiding estimation of the parameter. In reality, there will often be multiple sources of evidence and the identification and synthesis of all the available evidence for all the parameters in the model is essential to appropriately estimate the model parameters and characterize the uncertainty surrounding their values (Ades *et al.* 2005).

The methods for evidence synthesis of treatment effect are well developed (Sutton *et al.* 2000) and in principle should be applied to all model parameters.

In practice, the effect measure is usually the focus of formal evidence synthesis in most economic modelling exercises to date (Cooper *et al.* 2005). At several points the need for comparison of all treatment alternatives has been emphasized and this will often necessitate indirect comparisons (even where head-to-head trials are available). Such indirect comparisons are necessary for a full comparison of all treatment options, but are always subject to an increased level of uncertainty, and will clearly effect estimates of uncertainty and the value of information. The correlation between parameters which results from this type of evidence synthesis can add to the computational burden of value-of-information analysis and restricts the way parameters can be grouped in EVPPI and EVSI calculations (see Chapters 6 and 7).

In principle, we should also reflect any additional uncertainty due to potential biases in the evidence, which may come from different types of study and/or suffer from publication bias. Similarly we should also attempt to model the exchangeability of the evidence available with the parameters required in the model, reflecting any additional uncertainty in our parameter estimates. Scenarios have been used to explore these issues of bias and exchangeability (see Chapter 6) in a very similar way to issues of structural uncertainty. However, as with structural uncertainty, it is more useful to reflect the additional uncertainty in our parameter estimates based on elicitation of priors and/or estimating the possible bias or exchangeability. The practical challenges associated with explicitly modelling the potential for bias as part of decision models is huge, and the role for experimental designs for minimizing bias, particularly in treatment effects, remains strong.

A very similar issue to exchangeability is the inclusion or exclusion of what are regarded as unrelated events from the evidence and the potential role of prior elicitation from experts. The cost-effectiveness of a treatment strategy and the value of information can be significantly affected by the inclusion (exclusion) of unrelated (related) events (see Chapter 6). Often there is considerable uncertainty about how observed effects on events, which are not believed to be connected to the treatments under consideration, should be dealt with. In such instances, elicitation of prior beliefs on the magnitude and extent of any potential treatment effects on these events may have an important role in integrating this additional uncertainty into the analysis.

Finally, in some cases it will be important to deal simultaneously with heterogeneity (variability by observed patient characteristics), variability (variability by unobserved characteristic) and uncertainty. It should be recognized that the analysis discussed in previous chapters has primarily focused on uncertainty and has appropriately dealt with heterogeneity by conditioning the analysis on observed patient characteristics. As our purpose is to identify the alternative with the greatest *expected* net-benefit, variability will not be important in many models. In some nonlinear model structures, however, variability as well as uncertainty will affect the expectations of cost, outcome and, therefore, net-benefit. In these circumstances the analysis must integrate both the variability in the parameter and the uncertainty in our estimate of its value.

8.3. **Issues specific to value-of-information analysis**

Although the key challenges are more general and relevant to estimating cost, effect and decision uncertainty, a number of issues specific to value-of-information analysis need to be addressed.

Estimating the effective population that may benefit from additional evidence requires an estimate of the time horizons for different technologies and clearly has a significant impact on the estimates of population EVPI and population EVSI. A number of approaches to estimating the time horizon and effective population have been taken in the value-of-information literature, including considering only the current population; arbitrary time horizons (10, 20 years, infinite) and threshold population values. In addition, empirically-based estimates of the time horizons for decisions in health exist and can be incorporated in the analysis. However, all these approaches implicitly use time horizon as a proxy for future changes in technologies, prices and information. It is possible to explicitly model these future changes. Such analysis shows that the value of information for the decision problem may increase or fall over time, but the value of information for the group of parameters that can be evaluated by current research tends to decline. Therefore, finite and infinite time horizons for the decision problem represent special cases (e.g. significant price shock or no changes respectively). By explicitly modelling future change it is also possible to inform the timing of research, specifically, whether the research should be conducted now or delayed if further technologies are expected to be developed. Of course, modelling future uncertain changes is challenging and it may be that the use of finite time horizons are a reasonable proxy for this more complex process.

The EVPI for each patient group is useful in identifying where research will be most valuable (see Chapter 6) and which type of patients should be enrolled in any future trial. However, it must be recognized that further evidence about one subgroup may inform other patient groups as well. The subgroup EVPI is therefore likely to be a lower bound on the value of conducting research on that subgroup alone. However, the summation of value of information across subgroups will overestimate the value of research for all patient groups together. What is required is to model the exchangeability between subgroups so that additional information about one generates value to others. This is also true of decision problems: additional evidence about one decision problem may also be useful in informing other decision problems for patients with different indications or even different clinical areas (e.g. using the same technology for a different indication). This is very similar to the subgroup problem and we must recognize that the value of information for one decision problem is likely to be the lower bound on the value of research. In principle, the value of information can be viewed at a system level (the whole allocation problem for the health care system). This means there is an overall cost of uncertainty (EVPI) surrounding the whole allocation problem, and the value of information about a particular technology can been seen as the EVPPI for the parameters relevant to that technology. In other words, what we have described as EVPI for the decision problem is really an EVPPI calculation when we place it in the context of the whole system.

Value-of-information analysis indicates the societal value of further research when decisions based on current, perfect or sample information are fully implemented. Although it is important to distinguish the value of information and the value of implementation (see Chapter 6), relatively little consideration has been given to incorporating the value of implementation within the same analytic framework. In a budget constrained health care system, the decision to invest in implementation strategies must be made alongside those regarding investment in health care services and further research. It is possible to present both the value of information and the value of implementation strategies separately but simultaneously. An upper bound on the value of adopting implementation strategies (expected value of perfect implementation) can be established with current information and with perfect information based on the methods described in Chapter 6. This can give an indication of where priorities for research, implementation or some combination of the two should lie (Fenwick *et al.* 2004).

The discussion throughout Chapter 6 and 7 has assumed that decisions to adopt or reject a technology are reversible with no sunk costs. That is, we can adopt now, conduct further research and then, as necessary, reverse this decision in the light of the new information. As noted in Chapter 5, however, if there are substantial sunk costs associated with adopting a technology, or even irreversibility of the decision, then it may be better to delay adoption while additional information is generated through research. One reason why we might anticipate sunk costs is the cost of implementation discussed above. It is possible to estimate the expected opportunity cost of delay (net-benefit forgone) and compare these costs of delay with the expected benefits (the expected sunk costs avoided). However, a more complete analysis of this issue maybe offered by real options analysis. While the current emphasis of this approach has been on financial options, in the form of various derivative securities, the methods have been extended to the evaluation of real assets (e.g. real estate, proposed environmental developments etc.). These have become known as real options. Despite its analytical appeal, the techniques of real options analysis have yet to be applied in practice in the evaluation of health care in any substantive manner (Palmer and Smith 2000).

There are, of course, many challenges when attempting to estimate costs and effects across a range of possible interventions, over a relevant time horizon and for specific patient groups, while attempting to represent fully the uncertainty surrounding the decision. The issues of interpretation of evidence, synthesis, potential bias, exchangeability and appropriate model structure have always been present in any informal and partial review of evidence. In fact, until quite recently, these challenging issues could be conveniently ignored by both policy makers, clinicians and analysts, while decision making was opaque and based on implicit criteria and unspecified 'weighing' of the evidence. These challenges must be faced as more explicit and transparent approaches to decision making are being taken. Indeed, one of the many advantages of a more transparent and explicit approach to decision making and the characterization of uncertainty, is that it exposes many important methodological issues previously avoided by presenting partial analyses which do not directly address the decisions which must be made in any health care system.

References

Ades, A. E., Sculpher, M. J., Sutton, A., Abrams, A., Cooper, N., Welton, N. *et al.* (2006) 'Bayesian methods for evidence synthesis in cost-effectiveness analysis', *PharmacoEconomics*, 24: 1–19.

Cooper, N. J., Coyle, D., Abrams, K. R., Mugford, M. and Sutton, A. J. (in press) 'Use of evidence in decision models: An appraisal of health technology assessments in the UK to date'. *Journal of Health Services Research and Policy*, 10: 245–250.

Draper, D. (1995) 'Assessment and propagation of model uncertainty', *Journal of the Royal Statistical Society, Series B*, 57: 45–97.

Fenwick, E., Claxton, K. and Sculpher, M. J. (2004) 'The value of implementation and the value of information: Combined and uneven development'. *Medical Decision Making*, 24: 6 (Abstract).

Ginnelly, L. and Claxton, K. (2005) 'Characterising structural uncertainty in decision analytic models: review and application of available methods'. *Medical Decision Making*, 25: 6 (Abstract).

O'Hagan, A., Stevenson, M. and Madan, J. S. (2005). 'Monte Carlo probabilistic sensitivity analysis for patient-level simulation models'. Sheffield Statistics Research Report 561/05. Sheffield, University of Sheffield.

Palmer, S. and Smith, P. C. (2000) 'Incorporating option values into the economic evaluation of health care technologies', *Journal of Health Economics*, 19: 755–766.

Stevenson, M. D., Oakley, J. and Chilcott, J. B. (2004) 'Gaussian process modelling in conjunction with individual patient simulation modelling: a case study describing the calculation of cost-effectiveness ratios for the treatment of established osteoporosis', *Medical Decision Making*, 24: 89–100.

Sutton, A. J., Abrams, K. R., Jones, D. R., Sheldon, T. A. and Song, F. (2000) *Methods for meta-analysis in medical research*. Wiley & Sons.

Index